# Praise for *The Sleep Lady®'s Gentle Newborn Sleep Guide*

"If you're a parent of a newborn struggling to find sleep solutions that are gentle, work, and don't leave you and your baby in tears—you've just found it! Kim West, The Sleep Lady, is *the* authority on gentle sleep training for children, and now she has a book specifically for newborns! As a holistic pediatrician, I will recommend this book to all my parents and parents-to-be! Kim provides simple, effective, evidence-based advice that is developmentally appropriate with month-by-month guidance that is gentle on baby and parent! Get this book NOW and lay the foundations for sleep success to help your baby thrive at any age!"

**—Elisa H. Song, MD, holistic pediatrician and founder of Healthy Kids Happy Kids**

"I will recommend this book to all my new parents. It's simple. It's clear. It's gentle. It just makes sense, and (most importantly) it WORKS. Plus, most books on newborns only talk about the baby . . . I love that this book includes the well-being of the caregivers, because they need sleep too!"

**—Ana-Maria Temple, MD, holistic pediatrician and coauthor of *Healthy Kids in an Unhealthy Word* and *Ending the Eczema Epidemic***

"If you're a parent of a newborn who values sleep AND a gentle, responsive parenting approach, this book is for you! Kim West (aka The Sleep Lady) offers practical tips that are empowering, relatable, well-researched, and founded upon many years of professional and real-life experience. This in-depth yet simple guide will support the sleep and emotional well-being of your entire family."

**—Mary Wilde, MD, integrative pediatrician, creator of Compassion Parenting & Resilience School, and mother of eight**

"While sleep seemed natural to my first baby, it seemed like a foreign concept to my second. I didn't know where to turn as cry-it-out was not for me, but I desperately needed sleep. Kim West's book was a life- and sanity-saver for our family, coaching me to coach my daughter to sleep FAST with a gentle, evidence-based approach. If you're struggling with getting your newborn (and yourself) quality sleep or expecting a newborn soon, *The Sleep Lady®'s Gentle Newborn Sleep Guide* should be at the top of your reading list."

**—Shannon Willett, creator of Parenting Products Guru and mother of two**

"Kim West offers a compassionate approach to sleep that meets tired parents where they are. Her book helps parents understand and respond to their baby at each stage of their early development. A valuable addition to any parent's toolkit."

**—Alison Escalante, MD, pediatrician and adjunct professor of pediatrics at Rush University**

The Sleep Lady®'s

# GENTLE NEWBORN SLEEP GUIDE

**Also by Kim West, MSW**

*The Sleep Lady®'s Good Night, Sleep Tight*
*Gentle Proven Solutions to Help Your Child Sleep Well and Wake Up Happy*

*The Good Night, Sleep Tight Workbook*

*The Good Night, Sleep Tight Workbook for Children with Special Needs*

The Sleep Lady®'s

# GENTLE NEWBORN SLEEP GUIDE

For Birth Through Five Months

Trusted Solutions for Getting You
and Your Baby **FAST to Sleep**
Without Leaving Them to Cry It Out

**KIM WEST, MSW,** and her Gentle Sleep Team

BenBella Books, Inc.
Dallas, TX

BenBella Books, Inc.
10440 N. Central Expressway
Suite 800
Dallas, TX 75231
benbellabooks.com
Send feedback to feedback@benbellabooks.com

*BenBella* is a federally registered trademark.

Printed in the United States of America
10 9 8 7 6 5 4 3 2 1

Library of Congress Control Number: 2022948066
ISBN 9781637741566 (trade paperback)
ISBN 9781637741573 (electronic)

Editing by Leah Wilson
Copyediting by Karen Wise
Proofreading by Kellie Doherty and Sarah Vostok
Indexing by WordCo.
Text design and composition by PerfecType, Nashville, TN
Cover design by Sarah Avinger
Cover image © iStock / selimaksan
Printed by Lake Book Manufacturing

Special discounts for bulk sales are available. Please contact bulkorders@benbellabooks.com.

*To my daughters . . .*

*For being unapologetically unique and beautiful and teaching me
to recognize and celebrate your individuality and temperament,
from birth to forever. Love you to the moon and back!*

# Contents

*Start Here* ........................................................... 1

*Meet My Gentle Sleep Team* ............................... 11

*How to Use This Book* ....................................... 17

Before Birth ...................................................... 27

Your Baby's First Month *(Birth to 4 Weeks)* ................... 51

Your Baby's Second Month *(4 to 8 Weeks)* ................ 117

Your Baby's Third Month *(8 to 12 Weeks)* ................ 157

Your Baby's Fourth Month *(12 to 16 Weeks)* ............ 193

Your Baby's Fifth Month *(16 to 20 Weeks)* ............ 235

What's Next? ..................................................... 291

*Appendix* ........................................................ 293

*Acknowledgments* ........................................... 297

*Notes* .............................................................. 299

*Index* ............................................................. 307

# Start Here

> I remember leaving the hospital . . . and thinking, "Wait. Are they
> going to let me just walk off with him? I don't know beans about
> babies! I don't have a license to do this. [We're] just amateurs."
> —Anne Tyler, *Breathing Lessons*

I will always remember my conversation with Jenna, a new mom.

"Having a baby was supposed to be the happiest time of my life, but I was miserable," she told me. "Our baby wouldn't stop crying and wouldn't go to sleep. I was exhausted. My breasts hurt. My husband and I didn't agree on anything, and we were hardly speaking to each other.

"I tried everything, and nothing worked. I felt like I was a bad mom who was getting it all wrong.

"When I was pregnant, I had visions of sitting in a rocking chair, singing lullabies to my baby. It was nothing like that. I didn't know if she had gas or colic or if I was swaddling her too tight or not tight enough. Breastfeeding was more difficult than I had ever imagined. It was just s-o-o frustrating.

"Then, I found you. And for the first time, my husband and I had answers that worked. We both agreed with your approach, so we were no longer at odds with each other and at each other's throats.

"I almost cried with relief that first time she slept for 6 hours straight.

"Thank you! It's not an overstatement to say you saved our marriage. And the best part of all is that being a mom is finally how I imagined and hoped it would be."

Jenna's story is just one of thousands I've heard over the years.

Most babies aren't naturally good sleepers. Many parents think that there are only two options to improve their baby's sleep: let them "cry it out" or just live with poor sleep for the foreseeable future. And often those who do plan to "cry it out" (usually at 6 months) are told there is *nothing* they can do to help their baby sleep in the meantime.

If there's anything I've learned in over 25 years of helping parents around the globe, it's that raising a baby—even a newborn—doesn't have to be a sleep-deprived nightmare. There's another option: *Baby-Led Sleep Shaping and Coaching*, a gentle approach that parents can use to first shape their baby's sleep and then, when developmentally appropriate (and according to their baby's unique temperament), coach their little one as they learn to fall asleep and stay asleep on their own.

I literally wrote the book on sleep for children 6 months to 6 years—*The Sleep Lady's Good Night Sleep Tight*. Now, I'm sharing my even gentler, modified approach for babies under 6 months. Even in the first 5 months, there are many small ways that you can help your baby sleep just a little bit better—and together, these can add up to significantly better sleep!

## SLEEP SHAPING, SLEEP COACHING, AND SLEEP TRAINING

Part of self-regulation is your baby's ability to filter out stimuli, plus manage their own behavior and emotions, in response to their surrounding environment—whether it is putting themselves to sleep, signaling to their parent that they are hungry, turning away from a loud person who is too close, or eventually crawling over to get a new toy because they're bored. And self-regulation is crucial for babies' ability to put themselves to sleep. But self-regulation isn't something babies are born with. It's something they learn over time.

You've probably heard the terms *sleep shaping*, *sleep coaching*, and/or *sleep training* tossed about when it comes to getting babies (and toddlers) to sleep well. Let me share some definitions so that we're all on the same page when we talk about Baby-Led Sleep Shaping and Baby-Led Sleep Coaching.

### Sleep Shaping

Sleep shaping is the process of supporting sleep with a parent or caregiver's help and a healthy sleep environment and practices. It is the approach I recommend for the first 3 to 5 months of a newborn's life.

A safe, sleep-friendly space is the foundation of effective sleep shaping. But sleep shaping also includes regulating a baby's morning wake time and night bedtime. It includes the various pre-bed routines you can put in place to let a baby know what to expect next: sleepytime! It sets the stage for learning to sleep independently when your baby is developmentally ready.

The world usually calls anything more than this *sleep training*. For what I do, however, I find the term *sleep coaching* much more accurate.

### Sleep Coaching

Sleep coaching is gently easing a baby into the sleep process, once they reach a developmentally appropriate age, by supporting them as they learn to put themselves to sleep. Like a coach in sports, you can teach, direct, and support your baby, but a coach doesn't *play* the game, and it's the same with sleep. Sleep coaching is built upon the foundation of sleep shaping and includes continuing to support your baby each night as they practice putting themselves to sleep, slowly doing less and less as they eventually master the skill themselves. It also includes tailoring your sleep coaching plan to accommodate your baby's unique temperament.

Under the traditional sleep training umbrella, you'll find the *extinction method* (also known as "cry it out") and the *graduated extinction method*. The extinction method involves putting a fully awake baby in a crib on their own and leaving the room with the idea that it will teach them to fall asleep on their own. The graduated extinction method adds timed intervals after which a parent can pop back into the baby's room to soothe or check on them when they are crying or fussing.

The origins of the extinction method go way back to the 1920s, when American psychologist Dr. John Watson proposed the concept of behaviorism, which states that a child is a blank canvas and any behavior they exhibit is caused by external stimuli and not related to their own internal thoughts or feelings.[1]

The practice of letting babies "cry it out"—leaving them alone all night with no feedings or "check-ins," as some American pediatricians recommend as early as 6 weeks—is based on the theory of behaviorism. The thought is that this teaches a baby that their crying doesn't get a response and that this "lesson" will lead the baby to modify their behavior (that is, they will no longer cry and simply go to sleep).

Unfortunately, this method and its behaviorism roots ignore several big factors:

- Babies are not blank slates: Every baby exhibits their own unique temperament that determines how they respond to their external environment.
- Young babies are not physically or mentally capable of self-soothing—they can't roll over or bring their hands to their mouth to suck their fingers—and the ability to self-soothe, at least at a basic level, is required for *all* humans to put themselves to sleep, no matter their age.
- A baby learns best when they are experiencing low levels of frustration: enough to motivate them, but not enough to dysregulate them. If they get too fussy, or are hysterically crying, they *can't* learn the new skills that would help them self-soothe.

I don't recommend the "cry it out" method for newborns because they are not developmentally ready to learn to put themselves to sleep independently—which means that the whole purpose of the method is lost on them. Also, all humans need to be in a calm state to be able to fall asleep, so letting a baby get into a state of hysterical crying (a dysregulated state) makes it almost impossible for them to fall asleep without assistance. Additionally, regular, prolonged hysterical crying (crying that can be recognized as a call for help) can lead to a baby's stress response system being negatively affected for life.[2]

Parents often share their fears that if they soothe their baby rather than letting them cry, they'll create "bad habits" that will be difficult to break in the future. I tell them not to worry about creating bad habits in the first 6 months. In her research on sleep interventions, Dr. Pamela Douglas found that sleep training during the early months does not decrease crying (or prevent sleep and behavioral problems) later in childhood. In fact, sometimes the opposite can happen: Crying can *increase* and breastfeeding might stop earlier.[3]

I've got some great tips for how to sleep shape and support your baby as they learn to sleep, starting right from birth, but I recommend waiting to gently sleep *coach* them until they are developmentally ready. I'll help you assess when that is, based on your baby's unique temperament and current capabilities and teach you the tools and techniques you need to create a strong foundation for future sleep success.

## HOW THE BOOK IS ORGANIZED

I've divided this book's chapters by month. You're welcome to jump straight to the month your baby is currently in and learn how to get them FAST to sleep (though I do recommend reading How to Use This Book first, for an overview of the gentle Baby-Led Sleep Shaping and Coaching process). In each chapter, you'll discover fascinating insights about the developmental phases your newborn is going through, which can help you understand why they're behaving the way they are and what they need to help them sleep that month.

Many parents tell my coaches and me how confused and overwhelmed they are because they keep getting conflicting advice about sleep. They also tell me they're anxious because they don't know what to do and who to believe, which compounds the problem. I realized that what was needed was an easy-to-remember, easy-to-apply approach people could trust.

The strategies and tactics that we teach our newborn parents are based on four main factors: *Feeding, Attachment, Soothing,* and *Temperament* (FAST), each of which forms a pillar in the foundation that supports a baby's sleep.

Addressing sleep alone at this age isn't enough! And not only do your baby's Feeding, Attachment, Soothing, and Temperament all affect their sleep, they affect each other as well.

### Feeding

If a baby isn't feeding well, I guarantee that they are not sleeping well. When it comes to feeding, just following the recommended guidelines for each age can do wonders to support daytime and nighttime sleep. But you'll also learn gentle modifications that can help with sleep shaping, and later on, feeding will play a significant role in your gentle sleep coaching plan.

### Attachment

German psychoanalyst Erik Erikson posited that humans go through eight stages of psychosocial development throughout their life. During the first 18 months, his theory says, babies are learning about trust.[4] Your baby is learning to trust that, when they call out for you to help them, you'll be there, and this trust is the foundation for what psychologists call attachment: the lasting bond between a parent and a child based on the child's trust that their needs will be provided for. It's amazing what a secure bond with your baby can do for sleep. It not only provides a feeling of safety and security for your baby but also sets the stage for you as a parent to better understand your baby's cues—which is core to learning how to soothe them.

### Soothing

Soothing is what helps your baby trust that you will be there to help them meet their needs. Soothing is how you help your little one become regulated when they are dysregulated—when they are crying and unhappy and (because they are still just a baby) unable to control their emotions. Soothing goes hand-in-hand first with "putting" your baby to sleep and then with teaching them how to fall asleep on their own.

When it comes to soothing, one of the biggest questions I hear is "Am I creating bad habits by responding to my baby too much?" My answer at this age is a resounding no! Your job is to help your baby get to a soothed state so that they know what it feels like. Once they've experienced this soothed state where "all is well," they'll want to get back there. When they become uncomfortable, they will cry for you to help them get to this state once again. As they grow older, they will start to develop self-soothing skills that will help them get there on their own, but in the meantime, soothing them is up to you. That's why each month includes a soothing section devoted to teaching a number of simple yet stellar age-specific soothing techniques.

### Temperament

Understanding your baby's temperament is key to understanding their unique sleep patterns and abilities when it comes to sleep—and to helping them learn to sleep better. Distinct temperaments respond differently to various soothing, sleep shaping, and sleep coaching techniques. Is your baby alert? Active? Passive? Happy? Fussy? You'll learn to work with your baby's unique temperament as you sleep shape and ultimately create the sleep coaching plan that is the best match for you and your baby.

Each month we'll start by putting our FAST foundation in place. Then, in Getting You and Your Baby to Sleep, we give you gentle age-appropriate practices that you can try with your baby to help them with both their nighttime and daytime sleep. We start with gentle sleep shaping, so that you have some tools that support your baby's sleep without relying on brain and body development that hasn't appeared yet. The tools are tailored to the skills your baby *does* have—which is why we call the process Baby-Led. Then, once your baby shows signs of being able to self-soothe, usually in the fourth or fifth month, we help you create a gentle sleep coaching plan, using my tried-and-true methods, that works with *your* baby's soothing preferences and temperament needs.

Finally, in Your Self-Care, we'll turn our attention to you, the parent. Other books don't include parents' well-being; they make it sound as if once you have the baby, it's all about the baby. We want to support the whole family because you all are connected to the little one who is joining you. Yes, your little one is your big focus in these first 5 months, but we show you how focusing on yourself can really make a difference in how you support their sleep.

When we soothe our babies before sleep, we are helping them regulate and teaching them what it feels like to be regulated, which is an important part of sleep shaping and sleep coaching. But self-regulation is important for us, too.

When you are well-regulated and calm, you are able to accomplish four key things:

- ✼ You are better able to interpret your baby's cues.
- ✼ You pass on your calm state to your baby. (Thanks to something called mirror neurons, when we are calm and self-regulated, it helps our babies self-regulate.[5] The more you model calm, the more you influence your baby's neural pathways toward calm.)
- ✼ You model self-regulation for your baby.
- ✼ You have the patience to stick with gentle and effective sleep shaping and coaching.

In the past decade, much has been learned about what happens to the brain in the postnatal period. Various hormone and brain changes can make self-care more challenging. In his book *The Postnatal Depletion Cure*, Dr. Oscar Serrallach explains how birth mothers' ability to multitask is temporarily adversely affected.[6] (And by the way, it is not just the birth mother who experiences these changes. Other caregivers do, too.) Their brains instinctively slow down to help them focus on their baby's subtle cues. This focused brain can be very helpful. It helps us slow down and better recognize our baby's cues and communications. But the decreased ability to multitask can leave us feeling like there is not enough time to do all the things we need to do—never mind worry about self-care. You will learn about these brain changes and why supporting yourself through them is so important.

The bottom line is that your ability to nurture your baby in all of the aspects that help sleep is directly related to your physical health, energy level, and mental health. We're all familiar with the analogy of putting on our own airplane oxygen masks first, and nowhere does this hold more truth than when we are taking care of another little human in their first few months of life. You'll hear from experts in self-care who make it their life's focus helping parents (in particular, birth mothers) support themselves and their self-regulation through their baby's first few months and get advice for actually incorporating it into your already busy life.

Throughout the book, I share insights and stories from my experience and from my Gentle Sleep Coaches. I've also included advice from a team of respected baby experts, so you can trust you're getting best practices and the most recent research.

Think of it this way: You have an entire vetted Gentle Sleep Village of experts helping you along the way—pediatricians, lactation consultants, and clinical psychologists, plus experts in nutrition, birth practices, adult sleep, attachment, temperament, infant development, meditation, and communication.

You'll also hear from real-life families, who were at their wit's end until they used our FAST to Sleep approach, and how it helped them create harmony, and sleep, in their home.

You'll hear from Emily, mother of 2-month-old Ryan, who found herself exhausted from nursing six to eight times a night, night after night. The information in this book taught her that, first of all, what she was experiencing was normal age-appropriate behavior, but also that it could be modified. Using our tried-and-true strategies and tactics, Emily gently changed Ryan's sleep schedule and learned to identify and respond to his cues so that his nights improved . . . all without sleep training. What a relief to have Ryan wake only a few times per night!

Ann will share her struggles with her daughter Sydney as she went through the 4-month sleep regression common to many babies, and the clear action plan (with options and flexibility) they used to get through this big developmental milestone.

Through it all, you'll learn how to be a baby detective, looking for signs, clues, and cues for why your baby may be acting the way they are in the moment. You'll learn to soothe and calm your baby in the way that works best for them—until they learn to do it themselves. My team and I will be here to validate you and your intuition as well as give you some step-by-step suggestions.

I know and love that families come in all shapes and sizes, and I wish to be as inclusive as possible. My aim is to share these tools and methods through an empowering lens so that you can determine what is best for you and your family.

Are you ready for some caregiver cheerleading? Are you ready to discover why your baby is doing what they're doing so it makes sense? Are you ready to get all family members on the same page to create a calm home environment and let everyone sleep better?

Once again, welcome. It is my sincere hope this book gives you everything you need to regain your confidence and create the quality of life you want for both you and your newborn . . . now, not someday.

May the advice, recommendations, and resources in this book help you and your baby get FAST to sleep, and may this special time be everything you want it to be and everything it deserves to be.

Sleep tight,

Kim West, MSW
*The Sleep Lady*

# Meet My Gentle Sleep Team

In my work, I regularly consult a number of trusted pediatricians, psychologists, and other specialists. You will hear from this team throughout the book. Here I will introduce my top certified Gentle Sleep Coaches, who are frequently quoted:

## GENTLE SLEEP COACHES

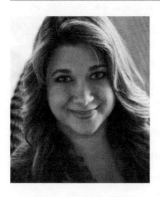

**Gentle Sleep Coach Heather Irvine, CLEC,** is an experienced mother of six children and highly sought-after infant consultant, parent educator, and pediatric sleep coach. Her background includes nearly 20 years of coaching and guiding exhausted and overwhelmed parents through the common challenges during the newborn stage and beyond. Her credentials include training and certification from renowned schools and organizations such as Harvard's Brazelton Institute, Healthy Children's Center for Breastfeeding, University of California—San Diego, University of Minnesota Infant Mental Health Department, and DONA. Heather has specialized training in areas of Newborn/Child Development and Behavior, Infant Mental Health, Postpartum Care, Lactation Counseling, and Pediatric Sleep. Over the years, her gentle baby tips and strategies have helped thousands of parents at home and virtually all over the world. Her company, Newborns & Beyond, is located in South Orange County, California, and offers infant consulting and sleep coaching programs to families of young children. Heather teaches the Gentle Sleep Coach 0–5 Month program.

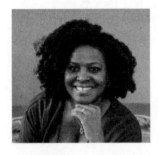

**Gentle Sleep Coach Brandi Jordan, MSW, IBCLC,** is a board-certified lactation consultant, certified Gentle Sleep Coach, newborn care specialist, and postpartum doula. She holds a BA in child development and a master's in social work from the University of Southern California. In 2009, she opened the Cradle Company, a pregnancy and postpartum resource center. Brandi's work as a consultant, parenting group leader, and in-home practitioner has led her to develop a unique philosophy of gentle parenting techniques that are a pragmatic, practical, and healthy approach for the whole family. In 2018, Brandi founded the National Association of Birth Workers of Color. Brandi teaches the Gentle Sleep Coach 0–5 Month program.

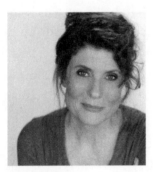

**Gentle Sleep Coach Macall Gordon, MA**, is a researcher, speaker, and author specializing in the link between temperament and sleep. Her research also calls for a more balanced take on sleep and sleep training. She has a master's degree in applied psychology from Antioch University and a BS in human biology from Stanford University. She is also a certified Gentle Sleep Coach in private practice as well as

*Joanna Degeneres*

with the women's telehealth platform Maven Clinic. She comes to this work because she had two sensitive, alert, intense children, and she didn't sleep for eighteen years.

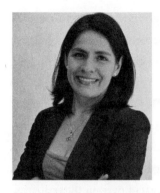

**Gentle Sleep Coach Gabriela Zepeda, MD,** is the founder of *"A soñar,"* the sleep coaching program of her comprehensive pediatrics practice in the south of Mexico City. Dr. Gaby is a mom, pediatrician, lactation counselor, and infectious disease specialist. She has a master's of science in pharmaceutical medicine and is a positive discipline parent educator. She also is an instructor in the Gentle Sleep Coach Certification Program in Spanish.

## MY GENTLE SLEEP VILLAGE

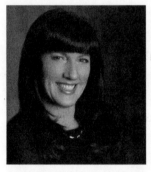

*Michael Benabib*

**Lindsey Biel, OTR/L**, is a pediatric occupational therapist with a private practice in New York City. She is coauthor of the award-winning *Raising a Sensory Smart Child: The Definitive Handbook for Helping Your Child with Sensory Processing Issues*, with a foreword by Temple Grandin, and the author of *Sensory Processing Challenges: Effective Clinical Work with Kids and Teens*. She is published widely in parenting and professional magazines and teaches workshops to parents, teachers, therapists, doctors, and other professionals across the country. Lindsey teaches the Gentle Sleep Coach Sensory Smart Sleep Strategies class (SensorySmarts.com) and is a faculty member of my Gentle Sleep Coach and Gentle Potty Coach programs.

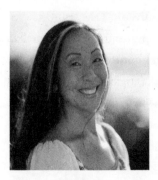

**Elisa Song, MD,** is an integrative pediatrician, pediatric functional medicine expert, and mother. Dr. Song has helped thousands of kids get to the root causes of their health concerns and has helped parents understand how to help their children thrive—body, mind, and spirit—by integrating conventional pediatrics with functional medicine, homeopathy, acupuncture, herbal medicine, and essential oils. She created Healthy

Kids Happy Kids (HealthyKidsHappyKids.com) as an online holistic pediatric care resource to help practitioners and parents bridge the gap between conventional and integrative pediatrics with an evidence-based, pediatrician-backed approach.

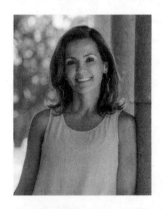

**Ana-Maria Temple, MD,** is a holistic pediatrician, bestselling author, award-winning speaker, and mother of three who has appeared on over a hundred TV news and podcast segments. During her 22-year career, Dr. Temple has treated over 36,000 patients. Her passion is to inspire, educate, and empower parents to revamp their family's health to prevent children from developing chronic disease. Learn more at IntegrativeHealthCarolinas.com.

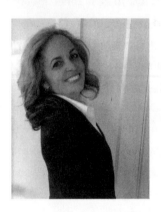

**Maryanne Tranter, PhD,** is an expert pediatric nurse practitioner, researcher, and parent mentor. She is the founder of the Healthy Child Concierge, where she helps parents with their anxieties about and worries for their children and works to resolve them. Dr. Maryanne has 25 years of experience caring for families dealing with colic. She also continues to care for patients in an elite pediatric hospital. Learn more at MaryanneTranter.com.

## YOUR SELF-CARE SUPPORT VILLAGE

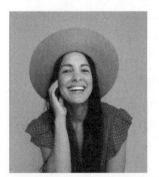

**Radha Agrawal** is an entrepreneur and cofounder, CEO, and Chief Community Architect of Daybreaker (Daybreaker.com), the global morning dance, music, and wellness movement. As a mother herself, Radha is passionate about practicing joy, finding community, and being present in motherhood.

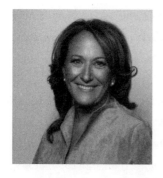

**Shoshana Bennett, PhD,** is a clinical psychologist and an expert on prenatal and postpartum depression and related mood and anxiety disorders. She is the author of the bestselling book *Postpartum Depression for Dummies*, as well as *Pregnant on Prozac* and *Children of the Depressed*, and coauthor of *Beyond the Blues*. Dr. Shosh helps us understand the difference between baby blues and postpartum depression by sharing what to ask yourself and symptoms to look for. Dr. Shosh is also a faculty member of my Gentle Sleep Coach certification program. Learn more at DrShosh.com.

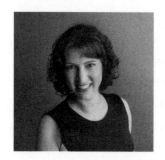

**Alison Escalante, MD,** is a pediatrician, speaker, writer, mother, and TEDx speaker. Dr. Escalante has reached hundreds of thousands of parents with her TEDx talk "The Should Storm." She is an expert in calm parenting and shares her parenting journey, including her mistakes, lessons, and ideas, at ShouldStorm.com.

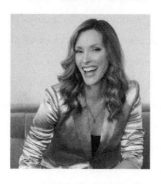

From a bestselling meditation book to helping Oscar, Grammy, and Emmy award winners, Navy SEALS, and NBA players learn to reduce stress and optimize their performance, **Emily Fletcher** has spent the past 10 years developing a unique and effective approach to mindfulness, meditation, and manifestation called the Ziva Technique. Emily is the founder of Ziva Meditation (ZivaMeditation.com) and zivaKIDS. Emily can help you tap into your inner happiness to become more balanced, whole, and emotionally agile and is an expert in mindfulness and meditation for kids. (Use code **sleeplady** to get 15 percent off any of Emily's online courses.)

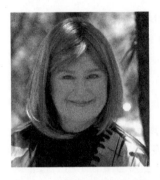

**Sam Horn** is the CEO of the Intrigue Agency, a communications consultancy that works with individuals and organizations to craft one-of-a-kind, respectful communications that add value for all involved. Her three TEDx talks and nine books (including *Tongue Fu!*, *What's Holding You Back*, and *SOMEDAY is Not a Day in the Week*) have been taught to clients at Oracle, Intel, Cisco, Fidelity, Boeing, and more. One of the great joys of Sam's life is helping people create first-of-their-kind books, businesses, presentations, and careers that scale their income and impact—for good.

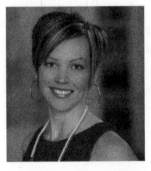

Certified parent coach and speaker **Samantha Moe** has guided parents on how to help their children calm, connect, and cooperate since 2004. She provides continuing education, advanced training, and parent coach certification for family service professionals who support intense kids and their families. Samantha is the creator of the Mad to Glad Blueprint, a revolutionary brain and nervous system–based approach to positive communication and parenting that works to soothe and even preempt intense kids' most challenging behaviors. Samantha holds a master's degree in communication disorders from the University of Minnesota and possesses a background in interdisciplinary training in sensory integration, play therapy, and emotional integration. Learn more at SamanthaMoe.com.

# How to Use This Book

**M**y Gentle Sleep Team knows that you'll have plenty of questions about your baby's sleep in their first 5 months. Your baby goes through many changes during this time, and your questions during the first month will be very different from your questions in month 5. This book is organized by your baby's age so that we can answer your age-specific questions—and so that you know right where to go to get the information you need as your baby grows.

Our decades of working directly with parents have taught us that the sleep techniques we teach are even more effective when parents know *why* they are effective. That's why we include specific information on development, feeding, attachment, soothing, and temperament for each month.

**You can start by reading the entire chapter related to your baby's specific age, but we suggest that you then flip back and read the previous chapters as well.** They will bolster your understanding of where your baby is now, as well as provide some valuable tools that are still useful in later months. Trust us as we guide you through this journey!

## DEVELOPMENT

All of our monthly recommendations are based on where your baby is estimated to be developmentally, so we start each chapter with an update on this. Please keep in mind that there is a lot of variability in the development of babies in the first 5 months. We share the milestones in order, but your baby might reach them earlier or later than other babies. Remember, it's not a race! Many parents worry about whether their baby is "on track" when it comes to development. Sometimes just knowing that the behaviors you see are common at a particular age can be helpful. We also encourage parents to trust their gut and get help from their pediatrician if they have concerns.

This section starts with the science, because knowing what skills your baby has helps you make informed decisions when it comes to their feeding, how to bond with them through attachment, how to soothe them, and how to interact with them based on their particular temperament. The section ends with suggestions to help keep your baby's development on track. There's a lot you can do! When your baby is growing and developing as your pediatrician expects, each month they learn new valuable skills that get them ready to both soothe themselves (with less and less help from you) and put themselves to sleep (yay!). We can't wait to get you and your baby to that point.

### Premature Babies

If your baby is premature, you can still follow most of the advice in this book. You'll just use your baby's adjusted age to determine which tools are most effective and when your baby is ready for gentle sleep coaching.

### Twins

If you are having twins . . . congratulations! While the advice in this book is written for singletons, it can also be applied to twins. For more detail on how to do so, check out my 2024 book with twin expert Natalie Diaz, CLC, CPST, *The Newborn Twin Sleep Guide*!

## WHAT IS FAST?

Great sleep doesn't just happen by accident. And that's actually lucky because it means there are things that you can do to help!

As we saw in Start Here, great sleep is supported by a strong FAST foundation: *Feeding* your baby, *Attachment* to your baby, *Soothing* your baby, and responding to your baby's *Temperament*. These aspects of your baby's life all affect each other and build on each other to support healthy sleep. When babies are first born, how well they sleep is particularly related to how well they are feeding. While you won't be able to sleep coach at this age, focusing on their feeding is one thing you can do to encourage better sleep. For example, if a baby is experiencing allergies due to something in their mother's milk, they may wake frequently at night from tummy aches or itchy eczema. Their parents may find them very difficult to soothe. Looking into the baby's nutrition and finding the source of the allergies may help them sleep longer and make them easier to soothe when they do wake. A strong attachment helps you better read your baby's feeding cues, as well as their soothing and sleep cues. Soothing is how we calm our babies and help them get ready for sleep, and temperament, too, can affect how easy a baby is to soothe. Some parents find that because of their baby's temperament, they need to do more to soothe their baby before sleep. It's all related!

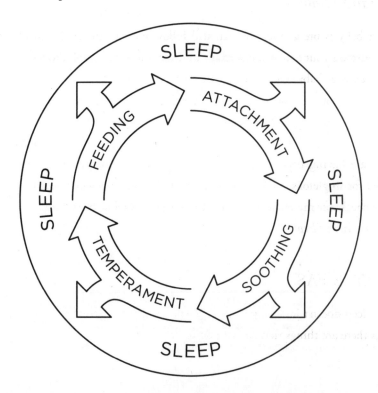

Strong practices in *Feeding, Attachment, Soothing,* and *Temperament* make for healthy baby sleep. That's why we've included sections devoted to each of these foundational areas of your baby's life. If you move the dial even a little bit in each of these areas, you can improve your chances of better sleep for both your baby and you!

## HOW TO SOAR

Your most important job is learning to read your baby's cues so that you can respond to them and meet their needs. This doesn't just reduce fussing and crying; the trust and bond you and your baby build as a result also ultimately supports their sleep.

Just because you now have a baby doesn't mean that you are magically able to understand them, however. Sometimes it will seem like they are speaking a foreign language . . . because they are! To make matters worse, they won't have figured out their *own* language yet.

I've got a four-step process to help you read (and learn) their cues and how to respond. It's called SOAR, which stands for *Stop, Observe, Assess,* and *Respond.* When you've got a fussy baby in your arms, sometimes it's helpful to have a tool to help you consider your next move.

You are your baby's detective, gathering clues to help you decipher their unique communication style. SOAR helps you look at each element of FAST to see what might be causing the fussiness or crying. It gives you concrete steps to take when you are unsure how to respond to your baby. It not only helps *in* the moment, but also builds your understanding of your baby's language so that you are more prepared the next time you are trying to figure out what your baby needs.

When you feel at a loss for how to help your little one, don't despair! It's time to SOAR!

When your baby gets upset, I recommend that you:

*Stop* . . . and take a breath. Holding a fussy baby can be stressful and make it harder to be aware of potential causes for that fussiness. Intentional breathing can calm you and bring you back to the present.

*Observe* . . . your baby's actions, vocalizations, and surroundings. What signals is your baby giving you? Are their arms and legs pulled in? Are they looking away? What are they doing with their body and their face? Is their diaper full? Are they extra warm or extra cool?

*Assess* . . . the current situation. What is your baby's current environment? What has occurred within the last several hours (or even the past 24)? Were there visitors? New smells, loud noises? How do the signals they're giving off correlate with their behavior, environment, and/or activities over the last few hours? You will learn cues that your baby may exhibit related to hunger, soothing needs, sleepiness, and their individual temperament, both from me and from observing your baby over time. Does your baby's signals correspond to any of the cues you've learned?

*Respond* . . . once you've determined the likely best action to meet your baby's needs. You might soothe them, quiet their environment, move to a dimly lit room to offer feeding or a diaper change, or assist them in going to sleep for a nap or the night. You will learn the next best course of action.

Remember, this is a process, and you are both learning how to communicate with each other! Using SOAR will help speed up that process.

##  GETTING YOU AND YOUR BABY TO SLEEP

In this section, we provide sleep averages and what you can realistically expect from your baby each month. We then dive into the developmentally appropriate tools that work best and share how to apply them. There are no one-size-fits-all solutions, so you'll read about options to try when both you and your baby are ready. You might be tempted to skip right to this section, but we encourage you to create a solid FAST foundation first, so that the sleep techniques we recommend can be as effective as possible.

In these sections, you'll also learn the elements that make up Baby-Led Sleep Shaping and Coaching. Sleep shaping sets the foundation so that you can gently and effectively sleep coach when your baby is ready. As you and your baby practice the sleep coaching techniques that you'll see in the following image, you will

# BABY-LED SLEEP SHAPING AND COACHING™

A gentle approach led by your baby's unique temperament and needs.

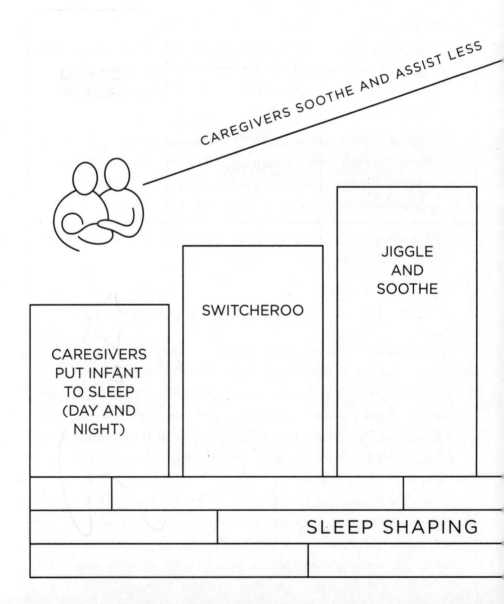

CAREGIVERS SOOTHE AND ASSIST LESS

JIGGLE AND SOOTHE

SWITCHEROO

CAREGIVERS PUT INFANT TO SLEEP (DAY AND NIGHT)

SLEEP SHAPING

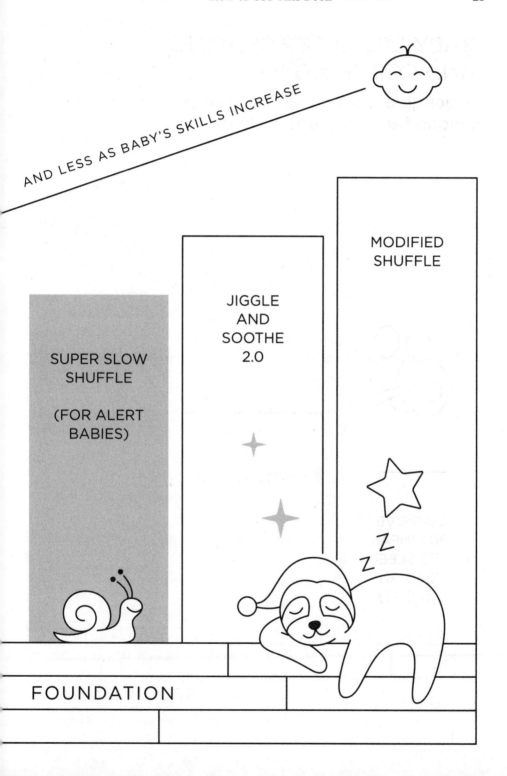

find your baby "doing more" while you are "doing less"—that is, as they learn self-soothing techniques, you will need to soothe them less and less.

## YOUR SELF-CARE

Speaking of skipping sections in chapters . . . don't skip this one!

I'm sure you've heard about the importance of supporting yourself during this time, but you might not have heard why. I've come to understand that **doubling down on your mental and physical health is directly connected to supporting the sleep needs of your baby**. Some of the reasons we share may be familiar to you, but others may be new, stemming from the latest scientific research. We've learned a lot in the past few years about how parents' minds and bodies change when their baby enters their world, and it holds true for birth parents as well as their partners and adoptive parents. This new understanding is both fascinating and empowering!

If *you* get restorative sleep, manage your stress levels, move your body regularly, and keep tabs on your mental health:

- ⭐ Your milk production can remain more consistent.
- ⭐ You will be better able to able to read your baby's cues and know how to soothe them.
- ⭐ You will be calmer, and it will be easier to calm your baby.
- ⭐ You'll have the energy to be more consistent as you implement our strategies and techniques.
- ⭐ You'll be more likely to recognize and experience the joy that comes with caring for your little one.
- ⭐ You'll have the energy to prepare to sleep coach your little one, whether on your own or with the support of a partner.

**By focusing on self-care, you are supporting the temporary brain rewiring that comes with being a parent (more on this in Month 1), and you're positively affecting your hormones and well-being.** All of this positively influences your ability to nurture your baby and effectively support their sleep. We've got some target suggestions that get to the root of mental and physical challenges you may be facing while making the most of your precious time. Taking care of yourself is not just for you; it's also important for your baby!

## READING THE FIRST 5 MONTHS

If you need to immediately address a specific sleep challenge, you can pop right to the month and/or subsection that will help you. But once you've learned a technique that can help, I highly recommend going back and reading the entire book, starting with Before Birth. We share many baby-related nuggets throughout that help support sleep from all different angles. For example, you may first zero in on a technique in Month 3 that helps you extend your baby's first stretch of night sleep. But after trying this solution, go back and start the book at the beginning—even though your baby may have passed some of the milestones we highlight. The techniques in earlier chapters can almost always be implemented later and will create a strong foundation for sleep coaching once your baby is developmentally ready.

# Before Birth

*As you await your baby's arrival, we'll help you prepare by sharing concept definitions that we will revisit throughout the book and guidance for designing your baby's sleeping area.*

A lot of this chapter is about *you*, and we want to talk about why *you* are so important. Other books make it sound as if once you have the baby, it's all about the baby. We want to support the whole family because you all are connected.

Self-care is not selfish, and it's helpful to put self-care habits in place before your baby arrives. Focusing on your own needs at this time will create a greater likelihood that you will be healthy and able to support your little one when they arrive.

 FEEDING

When we look at feeding in future chapters, we'll refer to your baby's feeding. But in this chapter, we're looking at *your* feeding—the nutrition your body needs to prepare and later care for your baby.

You're not yet breastfeeding or bottle-feeding your baby, but if you are a birth mother, you are providing both your baby (and yourself!) much-needed nutrition at this stage. If you plan to nurse, you'll want to keep your nutrition strong as you become a new parent. Your baby's feeding is one of the pillars that will support their sleep. If you won't be nursing, you'll still want to keep your nutrition strong, because a healthy diet will give you energy and more restorative sleep.

Shoshana Bennett, PhD, a clinical psychologist and expert on perinatal or postpartum mood and anxiety disorders (PMADs), shares that both sleep and nutrition are important to help prevent PMADs, particularly if you are at risk. For Dr. Shosh's wellness plan, which you can follow through pregnancy and postnatally to help prevent PMADs, check out DrShosh.com/WellnessPlan.

Holistic pediatrician Ana-Maria Temple suggests that we can best support ourselves and our babies with a diet that is healthy for the whole family. She shares that our gut has a very close relationship with our brain via the "gut-brain axis." The microorganisms in our gut influence our mood, appetite, stress level, and more. So, the better our diet, the better we feel both physically and mentally. For Dr. Temple's food and supplement recommendations, please see Shop.DrAnaMaria.com.

---

### Preparing for Your Baby's Arrival

The final months before your baby arrives are your chance to gather any items you'd like to have at the ready to help you nurture your baby's sleep. You won't need as many new products as you think! See our recommendations for "must haves" at SleepLady.com/Products.

---

 ATTACHMENT

Attachment is a deep and durable emotional link that connects you to your baby and is developed by tuning in to your baby's cues and responding appropriately to their needs. This special parent-child bond—created by a balance between the security that comes with support and the confidence that comes with being allowed to explore—forms over time as the two of you get to know each other.

Dr. Shosh suggests that we be aware of our relationship with our own caregivers when we were young—our attachment history—and how we might want to make our relationship with our baby different. If you'd like to do things differently with your baby, keep in mind that just deciding to do so isn't enough. You'll want to make a concerted effort: taking parenting classes, learning new skills, and, if needed, engaging in emotional work with a qualified therapist. Parents often need to practice holding, comforting, and engaging with their babies, especially if they, as children, didn't receive this type of nurturing.

According to neuropsychiatrist Daniel Siegel, author of *The Yes Brain* and other parenting books, changing our behavior also requires being aware of our own internal states (our moods) so that we can modify them and not parent reactively. This awareness allows us to connect with our children. It is often referred to as "parenting with presence."

Acknowledging our own feelings now is practice for acknowledging our babies' feelings in the future—and acknowledging and responding to our baby's feelings is the foundation of a strong parent-child attachment that supports healthy sleep.

## Bonding with Your Baby

The bond between you and your baby is essential to their mental development. But did you know that bonding with your baby can start during pregnancy or while waiting for adoption? For birth mothers, the maternal-fetal attachment forms as soon as pregnancy starts, but adoptive parents also begin to create a bond with their baby as they imagine what their baby will be like. As we wonder how our baby will look and what their personality will be, and envision what kind of adult they will grow up to be, that bond is strengthened.

If you are pregnant, you can add to this attachment by speaking to your baby in utero (the baby will then be familiar with your voice after birth!). And encouraging other family members to do so will help them bond with the baby as well.

## Learning to SOAR!

We introduce the SOAR process on page 20. You'll notice that the steps involved look at your baby, the environment, and the events around you, but an important part of SOAR is *you*!

When you Stop and breathe, you center yourself and set the stage for effective self-regulation. Being in the moment and "parenting with presence" allows you to better read your own internal state as well as your baby's cues and communication. It's important to not only observe and assess what is going on around you but also observe and assess yourself. How are you feeling? Do you feel centered and calm? Or stressed and on edge? How you feel affects how you respond to your baby.

When your baby is first born, they are operating from their primitive brain and relying on you to respond to them and meet their needs, since they no longer have 24-7 feeding and are no longer surrounded by darkness, warmth, and a comforting heartbeat (more on this in the next chapter).

 ## SOOTHING

Part of the attachment and bonding process involves soothing your newborn when they get fussy. Your baby is learning what it feels like to be *dysregulated* and then what it feels like to be *regulated* through soothing (as you learned in Start Here).

In the Baby-Led Sleep Shaping and Coaching process, for the first several months *you* will be doing the soothing, but in the future, your baby will learn to self-soothe and, eventually, self-regulate. Soothing is the first step to getting your baby to sleep at this stage. An upset baby is not calm enough to be lulled to sleep. Learning which soothing techniques work best for your baby will help you more easily get your baby to sleep.

# A Note on Trauma

Trauma is very personal—what is traumatic to one person might not be to another. Dr. Shosh points out, "Up to 6 percent of new mothers report having experienced trauma during the delivery. It is not what happens that causes trauma. Rather, it is how a situation or event is perceived that affects the psychological outcome. For instance, a woman who hemorrhages in the delivery room might not be traumatized if she feels safe, but a woman whose partner leaves the room for a minute might be if she is fearful she's been abandoned and is now alone and unsupported."

A birth mother might also experience post-traumatic stress disorder following birth. Dr. Shosh shares that the mother might have flashbacks, nightmares, insomnia, problems leaving her baby with anyone, and intense anxiety.

Dr. Shosh says, "When a baby's primary caretaker—usually the mother—is suffering from this condition, it can easily affect the baby and the relationship between them. If she doesn't receive timely help, she usually develops postpartum depression in addition. Babies with depressed and anxious mothers can be more irritable, harder to soothe, slower to develop motor and language skills, and eventually exhibit behavioral and psychological issues."

The mother isn't the only one who can experience trauma during childbirth. I've seen plenty of newborns whose sleep challenges can be directly correlated to a challenging birth. Taking care of your own mental and physical health will keep you better able to soothe your baby through potential trauma at this young age (you'll want to get professional help for this work). You will form a stronger attachment and be more attuned your little one's needs, so they can get quality sleep. You will also get better sleep yourself! And healthy sleep, whether for you or your newborn, is a form of healing in itself.

It is also important to learn to soothe yourself. Now is your chance to start paying attention to what dysregulation and regulation feel like. You can brainstorm activities that will help bring you back to your "happy set point" once you are a parent and start practicing them now.

 ## TEMPERAMENT

**Temperament is a hard-wired system for taking in, processing, and reacting to the internal and external world.** That said, a baby's temperament emerges slowly throughout their first 3 or 4 months of life and becomes clearer the older they get. Learning, recognizing, and working with your baby's particular temperament will help you know how to quickly soothe them and help them stay regulated in preparation for sleep. It will also help you understand their particular sleep patterns.

Babies who are more alert (see box) and who have more intense temperaments have difficulty filtering what comes in and have stronger reactions to it. You may find that these babies are also more cautious and introverted.

In *Temperament Tools: Working with Your Child's Inborn Traits*, pediatric nurse Helen Neville tells us that at one time, researchers (like Dr. John Watson, the father of behaviorism) believed all babies were born the same, and that it was

---

### Alert Babies

What I call "alert" babies (who later become alert children) are ones that are keenly aware of their surroundings, active, intense, and highly sensitive to both internal and external stimuli. Often, they are more difficult to read—it's hard to tell if they are "saying" they are hungry, tired, or in need of a diaper change. They can be more sensitive to transitions and, when they get older, often do better with a particularly gentle and slow approach to sleep coaching. Throughout my career as a sleep coach, 75 percent of the babies I work with have been alert babies—because those are the babies that are often in need of my help!

parenting style that caused babies to form their particular temperaments. Newer research proves, however, what many of us as parents already knew: Babies are born with their own temperament, and while that temperament can be highly influenced by events and caregivers, it stays consistent over the child's lifetime. Genetics appear to be responsible for between 20 and 60 percent of temperament. Interestingly, the sub-trait of soothability—how easy or difficult a baby is to soothe—shows no genetic basis.[7]

One landmark study from 1956 that tracked people from infancy to adulthood identified nine temperament characteristics that describe a child's behavioral style:[8]

1. *Activity level*: how active your baby is on a regular basis.
2. *Rhythmicity*: how regular or predictable your infant's sleep needs, hunger, and elimination are.
3. *Approach/withdrawal*: your infant's initial reaction to something new.
4. *Adaptability*: how easily your child adjusts to new circumstances or a change in routines.
5. *Intensity*: how strong your infant's response is to internal and external stimuli (both pleasant and unpleasant).
6. *Mood*: whether your baby is generally upbeat, serious, or somewhere in between.
7. *Persistence*: how long your infant engages in activity.
8. *Distractibility*: how easily your baby is distracted by external events.
9. *Sensory threshold*: the level of sensory input your child detects and responds to.

## Fantasy Temperament

You may have a fantasy about the type of temperament your baby will have. Perhaps you are quiet and introverted and unconsciously assume (or hope) that your baby will be the same. It's fun to speculate what your baby will be like, but it's helpful not to get overly attached to the idea of a particular temperament. Releasing expectations can actually help you bond more easily with your baby because you are more focused on who your baby actually is. Being open to "whoever you get," as I like to say, can really help ease your baby into the world.

## Goodness of Fit

**"Goodness of fit" is the level of compatibility between your baby's temperament, their caregivers' temperament, and their surrounding environment.**
When your baby arrives, you may find that their temperament fits well both with your own and with their surroundings. Or you may find that you need to modify their environment and even change how you might normally act in order to better support their temperament.

Before you meet your baby, it is helpful to get to know your own temperament. For example, how sensitive are you to crying and noises? Does change bother you? Your understanding of your temperament (and your partner's) will help you better relate to and understand your baby, as well as your own reactions and feelings toward your baby.

## SLEEP

As you approach your baby's birth, we recommend you focus on getting a good amount of sleep yourself, setting up a sleep-friendly nursery or other sleeping area, and preparing for sleep disruptions.

## A Sleep-Friendly Environment

A healthy and safe sleep environment is calm and comforting and not overstimulating and noisy. First, make sure that the setup is safe—you can check with your birthing and baby care class teacher for specifics on baby safety.

We find that most younger babies can often sleep anywhere during the day, but they might sleep best in their individual sleep space at night. The sleep environment that your child needs will be based on their individual temperament, so you may have to experiment a bit to find the environment that best fits them.

Our suggestions for a sleep-friendly space:

- ✩ A soothing room color, decorations, and fixtures.
- ✩ Room-darkening shades, if the room has bright sunshine streaming in during the early morning, naps, and/or bedtime.
- ✩ A dim night light. When you're feeding and caring for your baby in the middle of the night, you'll want enough light to see what you're

doing—particularly if you're changing a diaper—but not so much light that it completely "wakes" the baby (or you!). A yellow or orange (low blue) light is ideal. You can experiment with turning the dim night light off while your baby sleeps and keeping it on to determine which works best for everyone involved.

☆ A white noise machine. I often recommend trying white noise with all babies, but it is a must for alert babies who need a little extra sleep support, as it can help to block out noises throughout the rest of the house. You'll learn more about white noise in Month 1. An alternative to white noise is quiet, calming music or lullabies, which work better for some babies at bedtime. Be ready to experiment.

My team and I recommend a few products that can assist you at SleepLady .com/Products.

---

## Thinking about Sleep Montessori-Style?

Montessori expert Jeanne-Marie Paynel shares that the Montessori method proposes starting from the beginning without a crib to respect both a baby's need for movement and the development of their visual sense.

The Montessori approach suggests creating a safe sleep area in the child's own room—usually, a floor bed. It is recommended that—space permitting—babies sleep in their own room as soon as it is safe in order to support the parents' relationship and to give the baby an independent space of their own. Some parents create this environment as a future sleep space for their baby and help them get familiar with it when they are born, even if they co-sleep or room share for the first few months.

If you are still healing after your baby is born and find it difficult to get down to a mattress on the floor, it's okay to use a crib or bassinet until you are ready to move up and down easily.

It's also okay to have a crib at home even if the baby will eventually sleep on a mat during naps at a Montessori school.

## Room Sharing

Room sharing is when a newborn sleeps on an independent sleep surface in the parent's room for easy access and safety. (This is not the same thing as bedsharing, which is discussed on page 38.) The American Academy of Pediatrics (AAP) recommends room sharing with your baby from birth to at least 6 months.

Having the baby in a crib right next to you, in a bassinet that you can reach over and touch, or in a "co-sleeper" that attaches to the side of your bed makes it easy to feed them at night without having to get up. You have the peace of mind of having your baby literally at your fingertips, but you don't have to worry about the safety challenges of bedsharing. For moms who have had C-sections and have difficulty getting up and moving around for the first few weeks, this setup can be particularly helpful.

You'll also want to consider a backup plan in case room sharing doesn't work well for either your baby or you. Perhaps you find that your baby is particularly sensitive to your partner's snoring, or you are unable to sleep because you pop up every time you hear your baby stir. Your backup plan may be moving the bassinet into another room and even having one parent sleep on a separate mattress next to it. Make sure you have discussed your room sharing plan with your partner and are making choices that support your family's well-being.

If you plan to room share, whether for the first few weeks or longer, you'll want to set up your space so that you don't make a lot of noise when you go to bed.

---

### Sudden Infant Death Syndrome (SIDS)

Sudden infant death syndrome (SIDS) is the unexplained death, usually during sleep, of a seemingly healthy baby within the first year. SIDS is also known as crib death because the newborn often dies in their crib.

The exact cause of SIDS is unknown, but it is thought to be related to an inability to get sufficient oxygen. Either the infant's access to air is blocked because of their position (on their stomach or too close to pillows or blankets), or their ability to breathe is hampered by deep sleep caused by the comfortable stomach position.

Although the exact cause is unknown, several recommendations correlate highly with prevention, and you'll see references to SIDS prevention regularly through the first several chapters of this book.

In 2022, the AAP stated that evidence shows sleeping in the parents' room on a separate, safe surface lowers the chance of SIDS by as much as 50 percent.

First Candle (FirstCandle.org), an organization devoted to reducing sudden infant deaths, shares their top ten recommendations:

1.  Always place baby on their back for every sleep time.
2.  Use a firm and flat sleep surface covered with a tight-fitting sheet.
3.  Keep soft objects and loose bedding out of baby's sleep area. There should be nothing in the sleep area but baby.
4.  Room sharing is safer than bedsharing.
5.  Breastfeed if possible. Breastfeeding is even more effective at protecting against SIDS if it is done exclusively (not combined with formula).
6.  Avoid smoke exposure and alcohol and drug use (even over-the-counter drugs) during pregnancy and after birth.
7.  Consider offering a pacifier at nap time and bedtime once breastfeeding is firmly established.
8.  When you get tired, put your baby down in a safe place: a crib, play yard, or bassinet.
9.  Practice supervised tummy time to build neck, arm, and shoulder muscles and get baby rocking, scooting, and crawling.
10. Attend all well-baby checkups and immunize baby on schedule.

If you usually watch TV or use a laptop or tablet in your bedroom, you'll want to do this outside the bedroom instead.

## Co-Sleeping

The topic of co-sleeping, or sharing a bed with your baby (some people call it *bed-sharing*), is hotly debated in the world of infant sleep. Remember, this is different from room sharing, which is just having the baby sleep in the same room.

The AAP and the U.S. Consumer Product Safety Commission (CPSC) have formally recommended against co-sleeping/bedsharing for a child under age 2 because of the increased risk of death or injury from suffocation, strangulation, or entrapment. However, according to one study, **60 percent of new parents co-sleep or share a bed with their baby in the first year of life.** Knowing that this is a reality, my team and I tailor our advice so that it can also be applied to safe co-sleeping environments. We also know that co-sleeping has many benefits.

In lieu of co-sleeping, many families use a "side car" or "co-sleeper" crib that can be placed right up against the parents' bed. It has rails and safety measures but allows the closeness that many babies (and parents) crave in the first several months.

If you do have your baby sleep in your bed, your co-sleeping setup *must* be safe. Your mattress must be firm, with no pillow top. You must keep the bed free of pillows and loose blankets. You and your partner must agree that this is the manner in which your newborn will sleep. And an infant should never be placed in bed with a sleeping adult who is not aware the infant is there.

James J. McKenna is a professor of biological anthropology and the director of the Mother-Baby Sleep Laboratory at the University of Notre Dame. He is famous for his advocacy of safe co-sleeping in the United States (where it is less common than elsewhere in the world). Through anthropological studies, Dr. McKenna found that parent and baby heart rates, brain waves, sleep states, oxygen levels, temperature, and breathing influence each other when they sleep near one another.[9]

In his book *Safe Infant Sleep,* Dr. McKenna suggests a safe co-sleeping setup with "parents who do not smoke, are sober, have chosen to bedshare, and are breastfeeding their baby. The bedframe has been completely removed and the mattress has been placed at the center of the room away from walls and furniture. Light blankets and firm, square pillows are being used. No older children, pets, or stuffed animals are in the bed."[10] (Dr. McKenna's sleeping environment recommendations, as you can see, differ slightly from First Candle's and ours.)

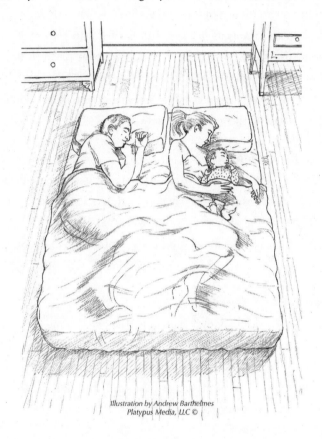

*Illustration by Andrew Barthelmes*
*Platypus Media, LLC ©*

(Note that the mattress is on the floor.)

British co-sleeping expert Helen Ball, BSc, MA, PhD, suggests that a nursing mother sleep on her side with her arm out above her baby's head (keeping pillows and blankets far away from the baby). This position allows the baby to nurse easily and safely at night.

I find that my co-sleeping parents fall into three main groups: Committed Co-Sleepers, Short-Term Co-Sleepers (the "We Started but Now Need to Transition" group), and Accidental Co-Sleepers.

### Committed Co-Sleepers

Some families decide before their little one is born that co-sleeping is right for them, and they set up their sleep space for safe co-sleeping. Once their baby arrives, everyone seems happy with the arrangement.

I encourage these families to eventually have their baby nap in a non-co-sleeping arrangement. This allows their nap plan to be longer-term and more sustainable, especially if they don't plan to co-sleep for a longer period of time. It will also keep the crib or bassinet from becoming a completely foreign location for the baby. Believe it or not, you will likely want the flexibility of having them nap separately one day!

### Short-Term Co-Sleepers

Some families think co-sleeping is for them, but once their baby arrives they find that it doesn't work for the baby or them. It is all okay! It's got to work for everyone. If you find after your baby arrives that you need to transition them out of your bed, you can check out my transition steps in the Sleep section of Month 5.

### Accidental Co-Sleepers

Some parents co-sleep out of desperation. The first few months of a baby's life can be a time of sleep deprivation for everyone, and parents end up co-sleeping because they are understandably doing the best that they can to get their baby and themselves to sleep. In this case, the baby has their own sleep space, but the parents bring the baby into their bed after particularly fussy periods throughout the night.

These co-sleepers need to be particularly careful that their sleep space is safe for their baby. I recommend creating a backup plan that allows you to co-sleep safely in case this happens to you. And if you find yourself in this camp once your baby comes and it is not working for you, I suggest you check out my transition steps in the Sleep section of Month 5.

Whichever option you choose, make sure that you have a plan and have considered the safety and overall well-being of your family.

## Reactive Co-Sleeping

If you're worried that you'll end up doing accidental co-sleeping, or what I also call "reactive co-sleeping," I recommend you create a backup plan. You'll want to make sure that you're not bringing the baby into your bed and accidentally falling asleep if your bed is not safe for co-sleeping. The same goes for feeding or nursing on a sofa and accidentally falling asleep.

One option is to put a futon or twin mattress on the floor of your baby's room for feeding during the night (follow the safe co-sleeping guidelines, of course). That way if you both fall asleep you don't have to worry about dropping your baby if you are in a rocker or having the baby fall off your chest if you're sitting on a couch. They also won't be in danger of suffocating in a bed with pillows, blankets, and quilts.

## Your Sleep

Try to get as much sleep as you can the month before your baby is due. It's great to get to bed consistently between 10 and 11 PM each night because you never know when your baby will arrive! Birth mothers regulate their babies' sleep in utero, so sticking to a healthy sleep schedule can benefit your baby, too.

Plus, sleep deprivation affects mood, cognitive ability, performance, health, and life satisfaction—every aspect of life. In her book *Sleep Deprived No More*, Dr. Jodi Mindell shares that it's not that different people have different sleep needs, it's that they tolerate sleep deprivation differently. You can't train your body to handle sleep deprivation—you either can or you can't.[11] I could not handle it well, which probably led me to become The Sleep Lady!

As you probably know, sleep problems are common in pregnancy. Studies suggest that these sleep changes might be caused by an increase in REM sleep (particularly in the third trimester) and a decrease in deep sleep. Plus, pregnant women can *feel* sleepier regardless of the amount of sleep they are getting because of the amount of progesterone in their bodies—and the fact that their bodies are taking care of two humans.

## Planning Your Nights

While you're pregnant or awaiting adoption, you can also start to think about what your nights might look like once your baby arrives and create a loose plan to support not only your baby but also you and your partner—so that you are getting enough sleep as well. After breastfeeding has been established, a nursing mother can express milk and have her partner, another family member, or a night nurse feed the baby when they wake so that she can get 5 or 6 hours of uninterrupted sleep. Another option is having one parent change the baby and bring them to the other parent, who then feeds them, reswaddles them, and puts them back to bed, thus divvying up the amount of time each parent has to be awake. (This division of labor can be especially helpful if Mom had a C-section.)

I encourage parents to take into account their personal sleep habits as they make their night plans. One parent might be a night owl while another caregiver might love waking at the crack of dawn.

---

### ☁ Sleep Lady Tip ☁

If you plan to return to work or to get outside help with the baby, it's never too early to start planning. This transition can affect a baby's sleep. However, we feel strongly that with a little extra planning and attention, it doesn't have to. If you're planning to return to work sometime in the next 5 months, please check out the appendix for tips for creating a transition plan that can support sleep—both yours and your baby's!

If you are at risk for PMADs, Dr. Shosh suggests that you make a plan now for how to get sleep when your baby arrives. The ideal is to get a minimum of 5 hours sleep in one stretch each night. If you're planning to breastfeed, you can work with a lactation consultant to develop a night plan that supports breastfeeding while still allowing you to get enough sleep (perhaps expressing milk so a partner can take over feeding at night).

## YOUR SELF-CARE

Sleep is, among other things, a form of self-care. It's a way of helping you self-regulate. But it's not the only form of self-care you should be focusing on as you await your baby's arrival.

Some self-care activities might be second nature to you. If you're stressed from a tough day at work, you might call a friend for support, go for a brisk walk, or practice some deep breathing to calm yourself. In the first several months of your baby's life, some of these actions might not be as available (if you're feeling stressed while trying to get your baby back to sleep in the middle of the night, it might not be the time to just pick up the phone and call a friend—though you'll wish you could!). You'll want to set yourself up for success by creating a self-care practice now that can sustain you and your regulation when you need it the most.

Your stress at this stage also affects your baby. Regular stress in the last trimester can cause birth mothers to release and pass on stress chemicals like cortisol.[12] Birth mothers who are particularly stressed may also have babies who, once born, cry more.[13] And a 2018 Canadian study linked prolonged maternal stress with the development of eczema in the baby after birth.[14]

Practicing self-care before the birth of your baby is also a chance to put solid healthy habits in place before the arrival of your little one temporarily turns your world upside down. So, we reached out to our favorite experts for ideas to help you take care of your mind, body, and spirit, which appear throughout the book. Here we've shared a few things to keep in mind as you await your baby.

## Prioritizing Your Health

Dr. Oscar Serrallach, author of *The Postnatal Depletion Cure: A Complete Guide to Rebuilding Your Health and Reclaiming Your Energy for Mothers of Newborns, Toddlers, and Young Children,* has studied the effect of pregnancy on women as well as how they recover after the baby is born. Because birth mothers provide the nutrition both for their growing babies and themselves during pregnancy, many become low in essential vitamins and minerals, and they can become depleted in other ways, too.

Dr. Serrallach suggests that they can replenish themselves with *nutrition, sleep, activity,* and *purpose.*[15] The more you can start focusing on these aspects of your life while you are still pregnant, the better off you'll be post-birth.

Holistic pediatrician Ana-Maria Temple advises the addition of omega-3s, organic vegetables, pasture-raised meat and eggs, and the vitamins and minerals that you can find in a complete prenatal vitamin.

## Creating Your Delivery Wish List

Many parents have a set idea of how things will go during their baby's birth. Some have their heart set on a water birth with a midwife, for example, while others look forward to the safety of a big hospital.

You may have been told to make a "birth plan," but as you've probably gathered from hearing other parents' birth stories, births rarely go according to a plan! Childbirth educator Amanda Gorman recommends that parents instead write down their birth *preferences*—that is, the aspects of the birthing process that are important to them. Thinking of this document as a list of preferences versus a plan will help you to be open to the birth going differently than you may have imagined.

I recommend opening yourself up to flexibility as much as possible. This mindset will help you during birth as well as afterward. We want you to be able to focus on supporting your little one's needs rather than being up at night worrying about what could or should have been because your baby's birth didn't go as planned. Remember, you are "in the club" no matter what happens during the birth process!

## Debunking Myths about Parenthood

As a clinical psychologist specializing in postpartum depression, Dr. Shosh knows a thing or two about the effect of parenting myths on PMADs. Being aware of these myths can go a long way toward protecting you from additional stress.

One of the biggest myths that can cause new mothers to head toward depression is believing that they should already know everything about how to take care of a baby. This attitude just sets you up for failure. Dr. Shosh and I agree that bonding happens over time. You might not instantly fall in love with your baby (another myth), and that's okay. It can take a while to feel a connection to your baby.

---

### ShouldStorms

Pediatrician Alison Escalante, MD, points out that as you care for your baby, it's not about doing everything exactly "right"; it's about creating a loving relationship. Surprisingly, even the best parents only get it "right" a third of the time. The problem is that most parents expect a higher "rate of success" and create what she calls a "ShouldStorm" of anxiety in their heads. ShouldStorms are what happen when thoughts about how we believe something should have happened swirl with thoughts about how we think we could have acted differently.

In her forthcoming book, *Sigh, See, Start,* Dr. Escalante goes into much more detail about her process for dismantling these ShouldStorms. It is in many ways similar to the SOAR process we recommend when you're trying to soothe your little one: Stop, Observe, Assess, Respond.

---

With sleep coaching, breastfeeding, and more, as with childbirth, try to remain flexible and open, and allow yourself to accept whatever happens. It's helpful to have wish lists for all of these, but know that you may have to think outside of the box in order to best support your baby and your family.

Please be gentle with yourself about your expectations and also what you think you "should" be doing as a parent.

## Handling Big Feelings

You may have heard other parents talk to their kids about "big feelings" (or if you already have a child or children, you may have used this phrase yourself). When you have a new baby, you may find yourself inundated with your own big feelings. New parents often find old memories and emotions, in particular from their own childhoods, surfacing at this time. And this is totally normal! The trick is to acknowledge these emotions while keeping them from interfering in how we care for and nurture our babies.

Especially if these emotions are related to abandonment, some new parents take this opportunity to explore these emotions further with the help of a trained therapist. But whether you choose therapy or not, there are other things you can do to support your emotional self and help yourself with self-regulation.

### Meditation

I know! You're thinking, *You're going to suggest that I meditate? With* what *extra time?* But hear me out.

Actually, let's hear from Ziva Meditation founder Emily Fletcher, whose company teaches the "Three Ms" for extraordinary performance: mindfulness, meditation, and manifesting.

Emily shares that daily meditation can make your brain faster and your intuition sharper—and help you sleep better. You'll learn next month about the changes that occur in birth parents', partners', and adoptive parents' brains; meditation is a tool you can use to support your brain through these changes. Your intuition is imperative at this stage as you lay the foundation for a strong attachment by learning to read your baby's cues and respond accordingly. And sleep . . . well, that's why you're here reading this book!

Emily likes to say that we don't have time *not* to meditate. She finds that meditation actually gives her more time. As she puts it, "We need to take meditation out of the 'pedicure for your brain' category and instead see it as our single most important piece of regular mental hygiene—something that we need to practice daily." Meditation helps you counter the stress that your body is feeling both in pregnancy and as a new parent—stress that manifests itself physically in your body through higher adrenaline and cortisol levels.

Some days you might choose to sacrifice sleep for meditation—and that's okay. (So is the reverse!) Meditation supports your brain and body in a different way than sleep. Emily shares that, when you meditate, your body is actually getting rest that is five times deeper than sleep.

During sleep, our breathing lengthens and deepens, highly oxygenating our blood. This allows our brain to safely go into "blackout sleep" while our body remains on guard enough that it may quickly rouse itself to fight or to flee from any predators that sneak up on us while we are at rest. The body is prepared for action while the mind rests.

During meditation, the opposite occurs. Our breathing slows and shallows. Our mind still has thoughts and our sense of hearing often becomes more sensitive, so that should we hear a predator approaching from afar, we can come out of meditation and oxygenate in time to fight or flee. Our brain is on guard while our body rests.

Meditation can also be used as a way to eradicate a lifetime of stress. Your thoughts are not the enemy. They can be seen as stressors leaving the nervous system.

Emily believes that meditation is actually the least selfish practice you can engage in as a parent. Because it replenishes your energy, it can positively affect your children, your relationship with your partner, and your interactions with everyone else in your life. In future months, Emily will share mindfulness exercises with you that you can easily incorporate into activities you are already doing with your baby.

## Joy Practice

In addition to nutrition and sleep, Dr. Serrallach suggests that a new parent needs both activity and a purpose to avoid postnatal depletion. Entrepreneur Radha Agrawal agrees. The company Radha cofounded, Daybreaker, helps others experience what she calls Joy Practice. Radha says that her Joy Practice is what supports her most in motherhood. She starts her morning looking for moments to experience joy throughout the day with a combination of dance, meditation, breathwork, yoga, EFT (a technique that involves tapping on acupressure spots), forest bathing (allowing the sights, sounds, and smells of nature to wash over you), and positive affirmations.

Recently, Daybreaker came out with a new offering called DOSE, which helps its members increase their happiness hormones (dopamine, oxytocin, serotonin, and endorphins) through a unique prescription of all of the activities she offers her Daybreaker+ members. (To learn more about Daybreaker, please see the QR code in Radha's bio on page 14.) These practices are in line with Dr. Temple's recommendations for activity and self-care as well.

According to Dr. Charles Zeanah, editor of the *Handbook of Infant Mental Health*, these hormones are integral to helping a parent create a strong attachment to their baby.[16] A delicate balance of these hormones supports a parent's mentalizing (their ability to understand their own emotional state as well as others'), empathy, and mirroring networks.[17] These networks in the brain are what help us be effective caregivers. So you can see how important it is to encourage production of these hormones!

In addition, Radha feels that much of parenting is about letting go and that the elements of her Joy Practice support her energy and presence as a parent.

What can you add to your day that brings you joy and elevates your mood? Start finding your own Joy Practice now and continue it postpartum to support both yourself and your baby.

Dr. Shosh recommends that all of her clients schedule a minimum of 2 hours a week for themselves. Go ahead and try to set up this time now and protect it even after your little one arrives—knowing that you have a block of "off duty" time to look forward to each week can do wonders in preventing burnout, depletion, and depression.

## ONE-PAGE FAST TO SLEEP SUMMARY

### *What to Focus on Pre-Birth*

1. Create your delivery wish list or list of birth preferences.
2. Consider how you might improve your nutrition to support your health.
3. Create a sleep-friendly and safe environment for your baby:
   - Decide with your partner where your baby will sleep (page 34).
   - Create a backup plan in case your initial plan doesn't work for your family.
4. Evaluate your own sleep and sleep environment (it's not too late to make changes!), and start going to bed at the same time each night.
5. Start your self-care practice: meditation, regular safe exercise, and/or Joy Practice (page 47).

For a printable PDF of this month's FAST to Sleep Summary plus helpful book bonuses, go to SleepLady.com/NewbornSleepGuide.

# Your Baby's First Month

## Birth to 4 Weeks

*This month, you'll learn about how your baby is operating from their primitive brain and about how you, as a parent, are experiencing brain changes that let you better care for your baby.*

When my daughter Carleigh was a newborn, she had mild jaundice. She was a "bird feeder"—one of those babies who eats small amounts and won't open their mouth wide enough to fully latch on—and breastfeeding was a big learning curve for the two of us. I was given well-intended advice from a lactation consultant to wake Carleigh during the night every hour and a half to feed her. The consultant implied that I had caused the jaundice by not feeding Carleigh frequently enough—and boy, did that make me feel horrible. I shared with her how difficult it was to wake Carleigh each time, and she suggested I strip her down and put a wet washcloth on her back (which seemed a bit mean to me) to wake her enough to feed.

Following this advice was a struggle. One night, I found myself all alone at 2 AM, crying, with a sleeping baby in my arms who wouldn't eat and a sleeping cat curled up by my side. I knew this feeding plan was not working for us. That was the exact moment I decided that I would follow my intuition (with the support of my pediatrician) when it came to how to care for my newborn.

I got up the next morning with a new directive.

I went against the social norm at the time by putting Carleigh on a flexible, gentle eating and sleeping routine during the day. I created a soothing bedtime routine and fed her at night only when she woke on her own—no more waking her to try to feed her. I tweaked, and I experimented.

I still wore her a lot and breastfed her (as was recommended), but I was following my heart and her cues when it came to when to feed her and how to care for her. I paid attention to her communication and responded to her needs.

In return, Carleigh was healthy and growing. She was happy and sleeping well (or as well as newborns sleep!). I was blossoming in my role as a mother.

I had the naysayers who said, "Oh, that's a stage . . . it will change" or "Oh, you were just lucky," and I would have my moments of doubt.

But I remember a nurse telling me, "That's not luck, Kim. It's you." And I kept that thought in my back pocket.

My experience with Carleigh taught me that the best thing I can do for you is encourage you to really get to know your newborn so that *you* are truly their expert. I want you to learn your baby's specific cues and unique personality so that you know how best to support them.

This is the first month with your newborn, so please don't worry if you can't yet recognize their cues. Learning to recognize cues is a process; it takes practice. You'll read more about what to look for throughout this chapter.

## WELCOME HOME!

This is an exciting time in your life! You have welcomed your newborn into the world and into your home. You're probably feeling excited but also a bit overwhelmed. My guess is that you are already feeling the effects of sleep deprivation and are wondering how to set your baby (and you) up for good restorative sleep both now and in the future.

I'll give you some tips and tricks on how to support your newborn's sleep this month, but at this stage, it's just as important to learn what your newborn is going through (both mentally and physically) in order to have realistic expectations. Knowing what your baby is capable of at this stage helps you understand that when your baby isn't sleeping 10 hours at a time (or achieving other milestones beyond their age), it doesn't mean you are failing as a parent.

# DEVELOPMENT

Knowing when your baby will reach a particular milestone helps you understand their behavior as well as how to soothe them. It also lets you know when to implement various aspects of sleep shaping. As I shared in Start Here, this gentle practice uses nighttime and daytime habits to lay a foundation for better sleep, so when your baby is ready they can more easily learn how to put themselves to sleep and *stay* asleep. Your baby will slowly learn how to do this over the next several months.

## *Developmental Expectations at This Age*

Baby's development milestones fall into four main categories: motor, sensory, communication, and feeding. This month we'll look at your baby's brain development and their automatic reflexes.

### Brain Development

It may surprise you to learn that most of the human brain develops after birth, not before. Babies are born with only 25 percent of their brains developed, and during the first year of life, their brains triple in size. **Ninety percent of all human brain growth occurs within the first five years of life.**[18]

According to certified parent coach Samantha Moe, humans have three brain regions: the *downstairs brain*, the *emotional brain*, and the *upstairs brain*, terms that were coined by neuropsychiatrist Daniel Siegel.

Samantha explains that the downstairs brain is responsible for the fight, flight, or freeze response and also the release of stress chemicals such as adrenaline and cortisol. As you might imagine, the emotional brain handles our emotions. The upstairs brain is in charge of solving problems, paying attention, and managing behaviors.

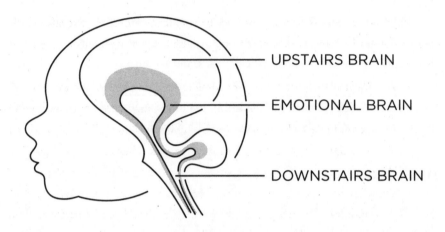

The downstairs brain is also known as the primitive or reptilian brain, because it is the most ancient region and has been largely unchanged by evolution. This part of the brain oversees instinctive behavior related to survival and controls essential bodily functions.[19]

At this stage, your baby's downstairs brain is all that is "online." Their upstairs brain, or neocortex, is unfinished.[20] In other words, your newborn is currently incapable of skills like imagination, problem-solving, reasoning, and reflection—skills that adults use every minute of every day.

That's why you, as a parent, are so important. Your newborn is unable to reason or determine how to calm themselves, so they need you to calm them.

Your job as caregiver is to learn and respond to your baby's instinctive behaviors, because these behaviors are really just requests for help. Your baby is looking for you to respond to their needs.

Your baby might be:

1. Hungry and need food.
2. Sitting in a wet or dirty diaper and need you to change them into a clean one.
3. Upset (perhaps because they are uncomfortable) and need your help to calm down.
4. Tired and need help falling asleep.
5. Overwhelmed by their new environment, which they don't understand, and need you to bring them to a quiet room.

Although one and two are obviously very important, they're also fairly straightforward. Three, four, and five require a bit more explanation and a few definitions.

As you learned in Start Here, when you're in a calm state, you are considered regulated. Self-regulation is the ability to monitor and keep your emotions in check. It is not a skill we are born with, but one children begin to learn around 3½ or 4 years old by watching their parents and caregivers. They take baby steps (pun intended!) as infants but are largely dependent on us to regulate them. Dysregulation occurs when you are unable to manage your emotions and, particularly, your emotional responses. When most adults find themselves dysregulated, they can quickly bring themselves back into a regulated state (often subconsciously—we might sigh when frustrated, for example, which is actually the body's way of taking a deep breath to calm ourselves down).

When your newborn gets dysregulated, your job is to help them get regulated because they are unable to get there on their own. Your response helps them in the moment, but it also helps them over the long term by creating a secure attachment where they feel safe, because they can trust you to respond to them. This "emotionally responsive" parenting helps your baby develop the crucial brain connections[21] that assist them in learning to successfully regulate themselves later in life.

You are also trying to help your baby learn the difference between what it feels like to be regulated and what it feels like to be dysregulated. Allowing them to become overly dysregulated by not responding to their needs can actually prevent them from learning and recognizing this difference. A baby (or any human, for that matter) in a dysregulated state cannot learn effectively. And this is a time when your baby needs to be learning an incredible number of new skills.

## Regaining Birth Weight

Babies typically lose about one-tenth of their birth weight in the first few days after birth,[22] but if their growth is on track, they will regain the weight and return to their birth weight within 2 weeks.

Note that an overly dysregulated baby can be very difficult to soothe back to a regulated state, which is why reading your baby's cues is important. The sooner you can come in with a soothing response, the easier they will be to soothe.

That's what's going on in your baby's brain. What's going on in their body?

## Newborn Reflexes

As the AAP shares in *Caring for Your Baby,* most of your baby's actions in the early months are reflexive—that is, involuntary. These amazing reflexes evolved to keep your baby safe while their brain is still developing. Some will remain for a few months, and others will go away in weeks.[23] It's helpful to understand what to expect regarding reflexes related to feeding and soothing in particular so that you'll know how to apply the tools I share later in this chapter:

| Reflex | Appears . . . | Disappears . . . |
|---|---|---|
| *Sucking*<br>The sucking reflex is a survival reflex that appears even before birth.[24] After birth, a baby automatically begins to suck whenever something, like a nipple, is placed in their mouth.[25]<br><br>A newborn may not yet be able to coordinate their sucking reflex while sleepy. You may need to wake them more completely if they are having trouble sucking (and then subsequently soothe them so they are calm enough to feed).[26] | Before birth | At 3 months |
| *Rooting*<br>This reflex begins when the side of the baby's cheek near the mouth is stroked or touched, causing the baby to turn their head in that direction.<br><br>Rooting, along with sucking and bringing their hands to their mouth, is a key feeding cue in the first weeks after birth. | At birth | At 4 months |

| *Moro (or startle)* | At birth | At 2 months |
|---|---|---|
| When your baby is startled by a loud noise, their head shifts position abruptly, or they feel as if they are falling, this reflex causes them to extend their arms, legs, and neck, then rapidly bring their arms together. This action may be accompanied by a loud cry.[27] Swaddling a baby to keep their arms close to their body can be very helpful to keep the Moro reflex from waking a startled newborn. | | |

These are some of the key reflexes your baby uses to communicate with you. You will learn to recognize these reflexes and understand how to respond to them.

## Crying

Between weeks 3 and 12, most babies go through a particularly fussy period due to a spurt in brain and physical development.[28] During this time, you may find that your newborn cries more than they used to, particularly toward the end of the day. This late-afternoon or early-evening fussiness is common for many babies as the stimulation that builds throughout the day becomes too much for them to process and handle.

If you can keep your baby from getting overwhelmed during the day, they'll be easier to put to sleep both for naps and in the evening. Stay tuned for the Soothing section on page 77, where you'll learn techniques to help calm them.

## Habituation

At this stage, your newborn has the ability to screen out sounds and overstimulating situations by going into a protective state called *habituation*. Habituation is one of your baby's rudimentary early coping skills.

When a baby is habituating, they appear to be sleeping deeply. They will often pull their arms and legs in and close their eyes. But in fact, they are spending a great amount of energy tuning out stimulation. You will find that there is no change in their respiratory rate, heart rate, or body tone. And while habituation isn't as stressful for babies as remaining awake, it *is* draining. A baby will typically "wake up" fussy, inconsolable, and exhausted after habituating, rather than refreshed and alert.[29]

Habituation might occur when a baby sleeps through dinner in a crowded restaurant or when they sleep through being handled by many relatives at a family function, seeming to be passed around easily. You'll learn more about how to recognize habituation and soothe your baby before they habituate in the Sleep section.

## The Fourth Trimester

As you know, many baby animals are born relatively independent, ready to move and run within hours of birth. Human babies, however, require all of their needs to be met externally for some time. We humans evolved to have large brains (inside large heads!) but also to walk upright (which requires narrow hips). This is not a great combination because the narrow hips don't allow a human mother to deliver a baby with a fully-formed brain. Therefore . . . **human babies come out a little early**, and continue their development outside the womb. This is why the first few months of a baby's life is often called the fourth trimester.

As they continue to develop, babies do best in a womb-like environment, and that's where your support comes in (see more in the Soothing section of this chapter).

## *Supporting Development for Better Sleep*

At this age, you have to do all of the soothing for your baby. Once they have the skills to soothe themselves even a little bit, they'll be able to calm themselves enough to fall asleep and eventually put themselves back to sleep when they wake in the middle of the night. But in the meantime, your job is to support them as they start to develop these skills. Babies learn best by experiencing these small bouts of frustration while you are right there with them, offering love and support.

One of the first stops on the self-soothing train is the ability to roll over, which allows baby to get into a more comfortable position. (Eventually, they will also be able to intentionally move their hand to their mouth and may choose to self-soothe in this way as well.) This ability doesn't occur overnight, but rather comes through the development of their core strength. And that means tummy time!

## Tummy Time

*Tummy time* is when you place your baby on their stomach on the floor to allow them to strengthen their core muscles through movement and attempting to lift and turn their head. The muscle tone and control your little one gains through tummy time is what eventually helps them change positions while sleeping, making them less likely to wake and cry out for help.

During the first month, my Gentle Sleep Team recommends **1- to 5-minute sessions of tummy time, 2 to 3 times per day**. Babies don't always like to be on their tummy because their head is so heavy at this age, but I suggest that you commit to this small amount of time if you can.

In the past, babies were regularly put to sleep on their stomachs, which meant that they were activating their core muscles a fair amount. Once we learned that sleeping on the back correlated with decreased potential for SIDS (please see page 36 for additional important information), babies no longer had the same amount of time on their stomachs. The result is that babies now, on average, learn to roll over later than they used to. You can help your baby roll when they are developmentally ready by committing to tummy time.

Tummy time is also when we first practice helping our babies learn something that might frustrate them a little. We practice letting them feel a bit of discomfort as they remain in a position that strengthens their muscles. This supported-learning dance will occur again when you start sleep shaping and sleep coaching your child. Practicing it now will get you both familiar with the process: You will get more comfortable with allowing your baby to feel healthy discomfort, and your baby will trust that they can handle small doses of discomfort while knowing that you are there to support them through it.

### ALTERNATIVE TUMMY TIME POSITIONS

Please don't despair if the standard tummy time position doesn't work for your baby. At this age, you can try a few alternatives to traditional tummy time that will still give your baby the core strength work that is important at this stage:

- ✴ Lying on a bed and putting your baby on their tummy on your chest.
- ✴ Holding your baby in a "football hold." (Use the palm of your hand to support your baby's neck and nestle them, on their side, closely against your side, tucking their feet and legs under your arm.)
- ✴ Doing tummy time on your lap.

The goal is to keep your baby from spending all their time positioned on their back with their head on the floor.

 ## FEEDING

We're going to focus a lot on feeding this month because it is the area of your baby's life that most affects sleep in the first month. Making sure that their feeding is on track goes a long way to helping your little one sleep. This section shares what "on track" means when it comes to breastmilk and/or formula intake and how to help your little one (and yourself) if you encounter challenges. And when we say *feeding*, we're talking about breastfeeding, bottle-feeding formula, and bottle-feeding breastmilk—any way that you are keeping your baby well nourished!

### Feeding at This Age

The World Health Organization suggests that parents practice exclusive breast-feeding from birth through 6 months.[30] I understand, however, that breastfeeding may simply not be an option for you. You have to do what works best for you and your baby. Your pediatrician is a great resource, and I support you in whatever you choose. You are here for your baby and supporting their needs, and that is what is most important!

### How Much Milk Should My Baby Be Getting?

It's helpful to remember that all babies are different—some like to snack often, while others drink more at one time and go longer between feedings. However, most babies will drink more and go longer between feedings as they grow bigger and their tummies can hold more milk.

## Average Breastmilk or Formula Intake Calculations

The daily amount of breastmilk or formula your baby needs is:

body weight (in pounds) multiplied
by 2.2 = number of ounces

For example, if you have a 7-pound baby . . .

7 × 2.2 = 15.4 ounces of milk or formula

Then, to figure out how much your baby should be getting each time they feed, divide this by the number of feedings.

So, a 7-pound baby eating 8 times a day should be having just under 2 ounces of milk or formula per feeding.

In the first month, most newborns eat **every 2 to 3 hours**, or **8 to 12 times every 24 hours**. Babies might take in only half an ounce per feeding for the first day or two of life, but after that, they will usually drink 1 to 2 ounces at each feeding. This amount usually increases to 2 to 4 ounces by 2 weeks of age.

Gentle Sleep Coach Brandi Jordan, MSW, IBCLC, recommends at this stage "8 or more in 24." That means that your baby is feeding 8 or more times within each 24-hour period.

## My Baby Seems Hungrier than Before

When your baby is born, their stomach is only the size of a cherry. At one week old, your baby's stomach has grown to the size of an egg, which means that they are capable of eating more at a feeding. In the week following, you may notice that your baby is acting "hungrier" than usual. That's normal! Most babies experience some type of growth spurt within the first few weeks of life.

## Feeding Is Going Well If . . .

✧　Baby is breastfeeding or feeding from a bottle 8 or more times within a 24-hour period (remember: "8 or more in 24").

✧　You can hear audible swallowing.

✧　Baby is urinating six or more times a day by 6 days old.

✧　A breastmilk-fed baby's poop is runny and liquidy, or a formula-fed baby's poop is the consistency of peanut butter.

## Supporting Sleep through Feeding

Since on-track feeding can really support sleep at this age, I have a number of suggestions for you on this front. The schedules and routines here may be counter to what you have heard, but I find that they work best when sleep is your goal.

### Should I Schedule Feedings?

You may be wondering if a schedule would help improve your baby's sleep at this age.

According to the AAP there is no need to feed your baby on a strict schedule at this stage unless your baby was born prematurely or has a medical condition where a feeding schedule is specifically prescribed by your doctor.[31] The World Health Organization agrees and recommends *on-demand* feeding instead (see page 63).[32] We are on board with this recommendation as well.

Although I don't suggest that you follow a schedule, you *may* see a rhythm appearing in your day. You'll see sleep and brief wake periods happening between each feeding that may look somewhat like the schedule below. (Because your baby's nap schedule may vary greatly, we've left out nap times and lengths.)

**7 AM:**　Feeding and diaper change (your baby will likely wake for the day around this time and be awake for only 45 minutes to 1 hour)

　　　　　Nap

**10 AM:**　Feeding and diaper change

　　　　　Nap

| 11 AM: | A good time for a walk |
| | Nap |
| 1 PM: | Feeding and diaper change |
| | Nap |
| 4 PM: | Feeding and diaper change |
| | Nap |
| 5 PM: | A good time for a walk |
| 6 PM: | Feeding and diaper change |
| | Nap |
| 9 PM: | Feeding and diaper change (your baby may go to bed around this time) |
| 12 AM: | Feeding and diaper change |
| 3 AM: | Feeding and diaper change |
| 5 AM: | Feeding and diaper change |

If you base your decisions on your child's rhythms instead of a strict schedule, taking notice of when your baby wants to feed, sleep, play, be held, burp, or tends to whine, you may discover a natural routine. That said, for babies with certain temperaments, no discernable routine will appear—so please don't feel like you are a poor parent if you're not seeing one.

If you do see a routine, be flexible with it as your baby's needs change! Enforcing a routine that has nothing to do with your baby's own rhythm is always going to be a struggle.

## On-Demand, Baby-Led, or Unrestricted Breastfeeding

*On-demand* feeding is when baby is fed as often as they want, day and night, whenever they show signs of readiness to eat. When breastfeeding, this also means that the baby stays on the breast until they come off on their own—usually slowing down with fewer sucks and longer pauses until they spit out the nipple and lie back looking content.[33]

Brandi points out that when breastfeeding, scheduled feeding can interfere with milk production (and, therefore, infant growth). A mother's milk production follows the needs of the baby, which are signaled by the frequency with which the baby nurses and the amount that the baby takes in. Scheduling feedings gives the mother's body a false sense of the baby's feeding needs, and her milk production can change accordingly—which can lead to potential feeding challenges down the road.

## Feeding and Sleep Logging

Many parents find it helpful to log their baby's feeding, sleep, mood, and diaper changes at this age. Even if you don't do this every day, a 4-day log can be very enlightening. It will help you to SOAR. You can look back and see when they last ate and how long they have been awake.

For example, you may discover a pattern where they get fussy every afternoon regardless of their sleep or feeding. I found this helpful with my daughter Carleigh. After looking at her logs, I discovered she would generally get fussy around 4 or 5 PM even though she was well napped and well fed. I would often take her for a walk around this time, and on days that she was particularly fussy, her dad would swaddle her, give her a pacifier, and put her in a carrier while I took some time to relax and get a break.

Check out my latest tracking app recommendation at SleepLady.com/Products.

Scheduled feeding can also interfere with your ability to read your newborn's natural feeding cues. When you spend a lot of time with your baby at your breast, you will begin to learn to differentiate their cries. You'll start to recognize their hungry cry versus them signaling the need for a diaper change or a nap.

The trick to giving your baby what they need when they need it is to pay attention to the time that elapses between feedings but not to specifically schedule feedings. This gives you an additional clue as to whether they are likely to be fussing due to hunger.

You can still keep track of when you feed your baby and for how long. In fact, we recommend it! Knowing that your baby has fed frequently over the previous few hours may help you determine whether the cries you hear are signaling hunger or instead some other need.

On-demand feeding doesn't mean that you automatically feed your newborn every time they cry. Remember to take a moment to SOAR:

- ✢ *Stop* and take a breath so that you are ready to focus on reading your baby's cues.
- ✢ *Observe* your baby's cries: Over time, you'll hear slight differences among them.
- ✢ *Assess* the situation: When did they last eat? Are they experiencing a growth spurt? How long have they been awake? What's going on in their environment? Does their diaper need changing? What else might they be trying to tell you?
- ✢ *Respond* with feeding or soothing as determined.

If you constantly respond by feeding your baby without assessing if they might have another need, you may miss the chance to help soothe them in other ways that better match that need.

## Should I Wake My Baby to Feed?

You'll hear conflicting advice on waking a baby to feed them. When they are this young, I recommend interrupting a baby's daytime sleep for feeding only if they go beyond 3 hours. The only exception to this recommendation is if the baby is already getting a solid eight or more feedings within that 24-hour window or if your pediatrician recommends it based on your baby's unique needs.

## Should I Introduce a Bottle Now?

The answer to this question varies.

When a baby starts attending daycare or being cared for by a nanny or other caregiver and is not used to feeding from a bottle, they can save all of their eating for when they are with a parent, which can disrupt both nap and nighttime sleep.

Some parents plan to transition their breastfed baby to a bottle when they head back to work. Others just want the flexibility of allowing others to feed the baby. Will your baby need to feed from a bottle within the next 2 months? If so,

# INTRODUCING A BOTTLE

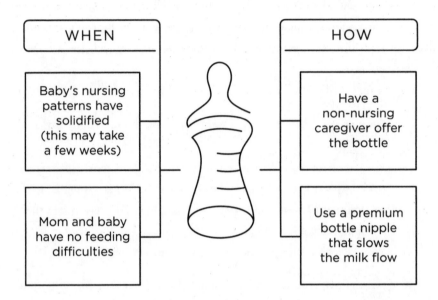

**WHEN**

Baby's nursing patterns have solidified (this may take a few weeks)

Mom and baby have no feeding difficulties

**HOW**

Have a non-nursing caregiver offer the bottle

Use a premium bottle nipple that slows the milk flow

Gentle Sleep Coach Gabriela Zepeda, MD, shares that now is an ideal time to speak to your lactation consultant so they can help you plan accordingly.

Dr. Gaby recommends that, ideally, a baby have 6 weeks of breastfeeding before a bottle is introduced, in order to avoid nipple confusion. The goal is to ensure breastfeeding is well established before introducing a bottle—meaning the baby easily latches on, breastfeeding is comfortable for the mother, and the baby is regularly gaining weight.

Timing is also important in reducing the likelihood of bottle refusal. If you wait to introduce a bottle beyond 8 weeks, babies have often gotten used to the breast and don't want to switch to something new.

## How Will I Recognize My Baby's Hunger Cues?

Hunger cues are present from the moment your baby is born. You'll see them in the first hour of birth, right before your baby feeds for the first time.

There are some universal cues that signify hunger in a newborn. Your baby is unique, however, and will have their own ways of communicating, as well as their own rhythm and style of feeding. Get your magnifying glass out and become your baby's detective.

Brandi shares that even though she has spent time with countless newborns, it still takes her 2 to 3 weeks to really recognize how each new client's baby communicates. For example, some babies like to eat more in the morning and not at night. Other babies eat slowly, while still others eat more quickly because Mom has a fast letdown.

Yes, a hungry baby often will cry. Their primal brain encourages them to cry to signal urgent needs. But crying is a late sign of hunger and can make it hard for a baby to settle down to eat, so it's best to watch for hunger cues before crying starts.

Typical early hunger cues include:

- ☆ Licking lips.
- ☆ Sticking out the tongue.
- ☆ Rooting (moving jaw and mouth or head in search of the breast or bottle).
- ☆ Putting hand to mouth repeatedly.
- ☆ Opening the mouth.
- ☆ Fussiness.
- ☆ Sucking on everything around.

Learning to recognize your baby's hunger cues helps you respond more quickly to their needs. A quick response reduces the need for additional soothing and will keep your baby from getting dysregulated, which requires even more soothing to help them return to a regulated state (and be able to feed!).

---

## Baby, Are You Hungry?

If your baby is fussing and you are not sure if they are hungry, the rooting reflex is your friend!

Put your baby near your breast or the bottle and stroke their cheek. If they turn toward and root for the breast or bottle, then they are hungry.

Using this tip in the first several months (until the rooting reflex fades) will help you differentiate your baby's hunger cry so that you know it when you hear it going forward.

It is important to remember, however, that crying or sucking does not always mean your baby is hungry. Babies suck not only from hunger but also for comfort, and it can be hard at first for parents to tell the difference. Sometimes, your baby just needs to be cuddled or changed.

As your baby's body and stomach grow, and they are able to eat less frequently, you can use your baby's cues to know the difference between hunger and other needs, and respond accordingly.

## Dunstan Baby Language's Hunger Cue

Dunstan Baby Language stems from the idea that a combination of natural reflex action and the pre-cry or cry sound coming from baby's mouth forms certain "words" that can be used to interpret baby's needs.[34] It's the brainchild of Priscilla Dunstan, who noticed patterns in her son's sounds that correlated to his various needs.

When a baby is hungry, they will start to suck. As they begin to cry, sound is added to the sucking reflex, and the combination of sucking and starting to cry sounds like the word "neh."[35] Louder crying makes the "neh" sound even more vocalized.

Please don't worry if you don't recognize this, or other "words" in the Dunstan Baby Language, right away. Learning them is a process and takes time. If you want to hear examples, please check out DunstanBaby.com.

## *Feeding Challenges*

As we've said, addressing any feeding challenges you encounter can really help your baby stay on track with sleep this month. Feeding is an integral part of sleep, particularly at this age.

## Breastfeeding Issues

Breastfeeding doesn't always come easily. If you're having challenges, please know that you are not alone.

Most breastfeeding issues arise within the first 2 weeks of life, and they can cause intense frustration for both Mom and baby. Whatever your breastfeeding challenge is—low milk supply, oversupply of milk, latching difficulty, mastitis—please know that there is usually a solution. Be sure to seek the advice of a professional lactation consultant at the earliest sign of an issue. You'll want someone who sees nursing babies day in and day out to help you both diagnose the issue and also share solutions.

## Allergies

Some babies exhibit allergic reactions to breastmilk, such as tummy troubles or skin reactions, that can keep them from sleeping well. Often what is actually happening is that they are reacting not to anything inherent to breastmilk itself, but to a particular food or drink their mother is taking in that is then getting converted into breastmilk. Dr. Elisa Song shares that the most common allergies babies experience are to cow's milk protein and soy. Gluten, corn, and eggs are the next most common allergies. If you think your baby might have a food allergy, be sure to consult with your pediatrician.

## Reflux and GERD

Most babies spit up, due to an immature digestive system. Usually, this is no cause for concern. Sometimes your baby may spit up from drinking too quickly, either from an overactive letdown or very full breasts when breastfeeding or, with a bottle-fed baby, a nipple that is flowing too fast. Your baby may also be swallowing a lot of air during the feed, which can also lead to milk coming back up.

Spitting up or regurgitation—often just called reflux—is common, reported in 40 to 65 percent of healthy infants. And although it may sometimes seem like their entire feeding comes back up afterward, looks can be deceiving, and odds are most of it has actually stayed down.

Gastroesophageal reflux disease, or GERD, is different. It occurs when the valve between the esophagus and the stomach allows contents of the stomach to regularly flow up and cause additional problems. It can be a big sleep disruptor! Please check with your pediatrician if you feel that your baby is spitting up significantly after feeding or if you're seeing any of the following behaviors:

☆   Vomiting after eating.
☆   Constant hiccups.
☆   Chronic irritability.
☆   Discomfort when lying on their back.
☆   Chronic cough and/or congestion.

There are a few things you can try to help care for your baby if they have GERD:

- ✩ Holding them upright for 30 minutes after feeding.

- ✩ Feeding them as a start to the day, rather than right before their first nap, and allowing for 30 minutes of upright play before they're put down to sleep.

- ✩ Offering smaller, more frequent feedings.

- ✩ Using the alternative tummy time positions that we suggested in the Development section (see page 59) to avoid additional pressure on their stomach.

- ✩ Nursing them, burping them, and then holding them upright as they fall asleep (rather than nursing them to sleep).

- ✩ Removing dairy from your diet or formula (when a breastfeeding mother drinks cow's milk, small amounts may end up in her breastmilk). Several studies have shown that breastfed infants with GERD may benefit from their mother cutting out both cow's milk and eggs.[36]

These babies will often feed for shorter periods of time during the day and then fuss after feeding but tend to do a little better with their nighttime feeds—perhaps because they are not awake enough to associate feeding with the pain that they experience afterward.

Babies with reflux might hold on to their middle-of-the-night feedings a bit longer than other babies—you'll want to work with your pediatrician before weaning them from their night feeding to make sure that they are getting enough nourishment during the day. (This is tough because your baby may want an extra feeding during the night to complete their nourishment for the day, and yet after they feed they are lying back down to sleep, which can make reflux worse.)

These babies may become temporarily dependent on being held upright to sleep—but please don't worry at this stage. It's important to get your baby the nutrients that they need—pain-free—and the sleep that they need any way you can.

## Supplementing with Formula at This Age

You may have heard that supplementing can help your baby sleep for longer stretches, particularly at night, but I don't recommend it solely for the purpose of longer sleep periods. Pediatrician Gabriela Zepeda says that supplementing for this purpose can lead to GI upset and may decrease breastmilk production. She says that there *are* appropriate times to supplement, though, and you and your pediatrician may decide that supplementing with formula is best for your newborn for other reasons. I encourage you to do whatever you need to do to keep your baby properly fed—especially since good nutrition will help your baby sleep!

 ## ATTACHMENT

Attachment—that deep and durable emotional link that connects you to your baby and is created by tuning in to your baby's cues and responding appropriately to their needs—is a major focus in the first months of your baby's life.

A securely attached baby is confident in their caregiver's ability to care for them and also their caregiver's availability: *They may not always be right next to me, but they will come when I call them.* Decades of research shows this type of attachment to have the best outcomes in a baby's physical, social, emotional, and cognitive development, in both the short and long term.[37]

A strong attachment will also help your baby feel safe and sleep better both now and in the future.

For more on attachment, please see our introduction to the topic in Before Birth.

---

### Attachment Parenting

I regularly remind my clients that *attachment theory* (and the concept of attachment) is not the same as *attachment parenting*. There is some overlap, however. Attachment parenting promotes the idea of feeding with love and respect, responding with sensitivity (particularly using touch and babywearing), and providing consistent and loving care. Physically and emotionally safe sleep is also a big tenet, as is striving for a healthy balance between personal and family life. My team and I are big fans of the principles of attachment parenting! To learn more, visit AttachmentParenting.org/Principles.

## Baby Bonding in the First Month

Some of us feel an intense bond with our babies the minute they're born. For many other parents, that passionate connection isn't immediate—and they feel guilty about it. Be kind to yourself; it often takes days or weeks to feel that bond, and it can even take a few months. This doesn't have to impact attachment. Secure attachment is the result of an ongoing process of positive give-and-take. It's about bonding *over time*.

Bonding with our babies comes from reading their cues, responding to them, and empathizing with their experiences. Your attachment tasks within the first month are fairly simple and straightforward. Your baby is looking for you to:

- ☆ Meet their needs by responding to their cries.
- ☆ Meet their needs by feeding them, changing their diapers, and providing shelter and emotional/physical safety.
- ☆ Let them regularly hear your voice.
- ☆ Make eye contact.
- ☆ Exhibit signs of affection.
- ☆ Provide nurturing touch.

These first few weeks, you'll spend a lot of time simply giving your baby attention and observing them. In these days of constant multitasking, this quiet time

---

### Eye Contact and Interaction

Shoshana Bennett, PhD, reminds us that our babies need eye contact and interaction with us because eye contact shows our babies that we are present and engaged with them, which helps them learn to regulate themselves.

The trick to effective engagement is to regularly display a wide range of facial expressions to your newborn. They are learning that your face is where they can look for a response.

Studies done regarding prolonged parental cell phone use have shown that it can have a negative effect on babies and children due to lack of interaction, as the "still face" a caregiver presents while using their phone can be surprisingly upsetting to babies and young children.[38] Both frequent disruptions (quickly answering texts/emails) and absorption (when a parent is fully engaged in the content on their phone) have been shown to be problematic—although I believe that absorption is worse, particularly if practiced for several hours at a time.

If possible, try to use your phone for long periods only when your baby naps. If you have to check your phone when you're with your little one, you can engage with them first, saying, "Sweetheart, I going to check something quickly." Your baby won't understand exactly what you've said but they will recognize that you engaged with them before your face went temporarily still.

It can be very gratifying to commit to moments of fully engaged interaction with your baby throughout the day. Think of it as a way to continue to bolster your baby's attachment.

with your newborn may actually feel a little boring and inactive. If that's how it feels . . . you're doing it right! This is your chance to learn to read your baby's cues, and for your baby to learn to read yours.

During this time, we want you to focus on your baby and yourself. And bonding with them and learning their cues is doing both. Learning your newborn's cues will allow you to respond to their fussiness more quickly and accurately—whether to simply calm them or help them learn to sleep. And this time investment now will pay off with more "me time" . . . and more sleep . . . later.

## Bonding with Your Baby for Better Sleep

Dr. Douglas Teti, a professor of psychology at Pennsylvania State University, has been conducting fascinating longitudinal work as part of the Study of Infants' Emergent Sleep Trajectories (yes, it's known as SIESTA). He used the Emotional Availability Scales—which measure parents' sensitivity and their ability to set appropriate limits, or conversely, their exhibitions of hostility when interacting with their child—to look at the correlation between emotional availability and sleep in 35 families with children ranging from 1 month to 2 years of age. It's probably not surprising that he found that "infants of mothers with high emotional availability had fewer bedtime disruptions and woke up less during the night."[39] I bet the same findings would be true for fathers, too.

Examples of emotional availability are parents cuddling and talking softly to their infants at bedtime and speaking reassuring phrases such as "It's okay" or "There, there" as they prepare them for sleep.

---

### Emotional Availability at Bedtime

The bedtime routine, in particular, is a lovely opportunity to connect and bond emotionally with your baby. I suggest not bringing a phone or tablet into your baby's sleep area and making time for kissing, hugging, and snuggling during the various steps in their soothing bedtime routine.

---

Dr. Teti's work has broader implications than **bedtime cuddling equals happy babies**. Emotional availability is about more than putting the baby to bed; it's about how we relate to our children overall. When we are fully present with our babies, they feel secure, and that helps them feel safe falling asleep—and staying asleep.

## Ways to Bond with Your Baby

Here are some of the easiest ways to nudge attachment along (some of which may be intuitive to you).

### Create Routines and Predictability

To feel safe and secure, babies need to know that they can count on you. Routines help meet this need for predictability, and thus are an important part of your baby's life. Routines let your baby learn *I know what's coming next*, which is comforting.

While in utero, everything in your baby's world was fairly simple and consistent. They were in a warm environment, fed constantly, and comforted by the soothing sound of Mom's heartbeat. Once born, they entered a world that was new and unfamiliar, filled with foreign sights, sounds, and smells. The more consistently you comfort your baby, the more safe and secure they are likely to feel.

We all have routines for our days. Most of us wake up in the morning and fall asleep at the end of the day at predictable times, work certain hours, eat around the same times every day. Routines bring structure to our lives, and structure and predictability help us feel secure. Putting routines in place for your baby will do the same and bring about positive benefits for your child and for your family as a whole.

You can begin to weave small routines into your days and evenings as early as your baby's third week. Start by taking a morning walk, practicing tummy time midday, reading to them in the afternoon, and/or giving them a nice warm bath and a massage in the evening before you put them down to bed.

Your goal is to create routines that your baby can expect and count on—and not just at bedtime, mealtime, and bath time. For example, you might have a special toy for diaper changes or a favorite song as you start your daily walk.

Bedtime routines can help your baby fall asleep faster and help defuse nighttime fussiness. Some babies fall into routines easily, while others may take some time to adjust. Believe it or not, it only takes a week (or less) for most young babies to acclimate to new routines.

### Four Areas Where You Can Build Routines

**Feeding**

Build some familiar routines around feeding. Some parents have a favorite chair they sit in while feeding their baby or use a special feeding pillow.

**Playtime**

Give your baby regular tummy time on the same blanket or play mat. Use this blanket or play mat around the same time every day.

**Naps**

Try to do the same two or three things prior to putting your baby down for each nap. These can be simple and quick, like singing a little lullaby and swaddling them.

**Bedtime**

Establish a few cozy and relaxing steps before putting your baby down for the night. Baths, books, and massage are all wonderful routines you can start early on.

Try not to get too caught up with rigid schedules or following the clock to the minute. But do try to set up a nice consistent flow to your day, where you do things in the same order on a regular basis. Babies typically sleep, eat, have a brief period of activity, and then begin to get tired again. You can use this natural cycle as your framework. Observe your baby's patterns to determine their natural flow and blend your routines in.

## Respond

Respond to your baby's needs promptly. No, you don't need to run; just let them know you heard them and will be there as soon as you can. This is an easy way to build a bond with your baby. If they cry because they are wet, changing them lets them know you've heard them. If they make hungry noises, feeding them teaches them what they need to feel better, and that you can be trusted to help. If you can't address their needs immediately, if possible, talk to them while you finish whatever you're doing (such as taking care of another child). You can't spoil your baby by being "too responsive" in the first few months of life.

## Hold Them!

Hug your baby, cuddle them, look into their eyes, and when they coo at you, coo back! Strap them onto your chest or use a sling rather than a stroller when it works for you. Sucking, touch, and warmth all release the calming chemical oxytocin in a baby's brain, which can bring down stress levels.[40]

On the other hand, you don't have to "wear" your baby every minute, and it's not a crime to use a bouncy seat some of the time. Remember that babies need and enjoy stimulation from baby gyms, tummy time, and the like, too, so you don't need to hold them all of the time.

## Kangaroo Care

*Kangaroo care* is a term for when a mother, father, or caregiver engages in extended skin-to-skin contact with the baby.[41] It is particularly helpful with low birth weight or premature babies, as it gives them the same benefits as an incubator and more— it's been shown to stabilize high-risk babies' breathing and heart rate, and reduce the risk of infection—but all newborns can benefit from kangaroo care.

For the mother, regular skin-to-skin contact supports both breastfeeding and bonding because it stimulates the release of helpful hormones, specifically prolactin and oxytocin, from the pituitary gland. It helps initiate breastfeeding earlier, which helps the baby gain weight faster. And it helps all parents and caregivers develop a close relationship with their baby.

To practice safe kangaroo care, place baby naked (except for a diaper for cleanliness and a cap to keep their head warm) in an upright position on the chest (for women, between the breasts). Support them in this position using clothes or other cloth tied around your chest, leaving their head free so that they can breathe unobstructed and making sure their face can be seen so you can read their cues.

 ## SOOTHING

Part of the attachment and bonding process is the act of soothing your newborn when they cry or get fussy. Eventually, you will learn to read their cues to understand exactly which need has to be met, but until then, there are some simple ways to soothe them and help them feel safe and secure.

Soothing is also the first step to getting your baby to sleep at this stage. Remember, an upset and dysregulated baby is not calm enough to be lulled to sleep.

Remember when you learned about your baby's current state of brain development? They are operating from their downstairs, or primal, brain, and their rage, fear, and separation distress systems are helping them stay safe.[42] It is not surprising that they become afraid after hearing a loud noise or get upset when you put them down after a cozy, warm snuggle. Your baby is genetically programmed to cry out for soothing when they are upset. Crying is their way of asking for help in easing frightening emotions and scary-at-times bodily sensations.[43]

As you know, I don't recommend letting a baby cry without attempting to soothe them. I want you to understand, however, that the crying itself does not negatively affect a baby's developing brain. What negatively affects the brain is *prolonged* unsoothed distress, which causes them to become especially dysregulated.[44]

Your baby will learn to self-regulate by experiencing and learning to handle short periods of frustration and light dysregulation. These experiences help them learn, but only if they are age-appropriate and overseen by a supportive caregiver. The problem is that we're often not told what is age-appropriate and what our babies can handle developmentally (this is why we include a Development section in each chapter). Frustration beyond a baby's developmental capacity leads to withdrawal behavior.[45] Withdrawal is not the same as independence. We are not looking for a quiet, independent baby at this age. Rather, withdrawal is a coping mechanism babies use when they experience regular dysregulation.

At this stage, we respond to our infants and soothe them because they are incapable of doing it themselves. This teaches them what it feels like to be soothed and regulated, which in turn helps them learn to self-soothe in the future. When

---

### ☁ Sleep Lady Tip ☁

Soothing is important both to comfort your baby in the moment and to support their healthy brain development for long-term growth and success.

they learn new self-soothing techniques in the future, they will repeat the ones that bring them to the regulated state they have learned to experience with your help.

Believe it or not, your continued regular response can keep your baby from exhibiting intense reactions to stress in the future. This comes from building trust. They learn to trust that their communication will be heard. If your baby knows that you'll respond to them in short order, they are less likely to overdo it on the crying or fussiness.

When your baby uses a cue that seems to work—when you respond to that cue by meeting the correct need—they will repeat it. As you see their cues repeat, it will get easier for you to recognize your newborn's needs. Soon, you will have your own special language with your baby. The more you respond to their cues, the faster they will learn which cues work best.

## Tips for Soothing Your Baby

Eventually, your baby will have many tools in their self-soothing toolbox that they can use to soothe themselves. For now, when you're in charge of soothing them, we're giving you a number of soothing tools to add to *your* soothing toolbox.

Remember that your baby was used to the womb environment, where the sound level was to their liking, they were warm and comfortable, and they had access to food when they needed it. Your job is to, as much as possible, replicate this environment and soothe them as they try to make sense of their new world. Sometimes close contact is enough to soothe them, but sometimes they need more.

Dr. Harvey Karp's popular book *The Happiest Baby on the Block: The New Way to Calm Crying and Help Your Newborn Baby Sleep Longer* recommends the "5 S's"—swaddling, side holding, "sh-sh-shing," swinging, and sucking—to get baby through the first few months.

 ### Swaddling

Swaddling is tightly wrapping your baby in a blanket to restrict the movement of their arms and legs. This is especially helpful at this stage due to the *Moro* or *startle*

*reflex*, where their arms and legs suddenly move involuntarily. This reflex occurs both when they are awake and asleep.

The pressure of swaddling, similar to what babies felt in utero, comforts them and can lengthen their sleep—and it often works well along with white noise (more on that shortly).

There are a lot of great swaddling products to choose from! Check out SleepLady.com/Products for my recommendations.

---

## How to Swaddle Safely

- Baby's legs and hips should not be wrapped so tightly as to completely restrict movement.
- Legs should be free to move up and out.
- Arms are bound firmly but not too tightly, either straight down next to their torso or bent across their chest.
- Avoid too much pressure on the chest.
- When swaddling your baby for sleep, *never* lay them down on their stomach. There is a high correlation between suffocation and babies who are swaddled and laid on their tummy to sleep.
- Be aware of their temperature and dress them accordingly—sometimes, just a diaper underneath is sufficient.
- Swaddle your baby only to calm them or for sleeping.
- Swaddling should be discontinued once your baby is rolling or close to doing so, to prevent them from rolling onto their stomach and getting stuck there, unable to breathe.

---

As simple as it may seem, swaddling does come with some risks. There are some safety concerns that every parent should be aware of if swaddling their baby, including suffocation, hip dysplasia, and overheating. However, if swaddling is done properly and safely, most of these risks can be avoided (see box).

Please keep in mind that while swaddling babies can be very helpful during sleep, it is not recommended that you swaddle your baby during their wakeful hours, as they need time to move and explore their world and environment.

### BENEFITS OF SWADDLING

If you are swaddling your baby safely, you may see the following benefits:

- ✧ Longer and deeper sleep. (Note that this is also a risk factor, as a baby in deep sleep may not awaken even if they get into an unsafe sleeping situation.)
- ✧ Less crying.
- ✧ Easier calming and soothing. (When your baby's arms are swaddled so that they cross their midline, their right- and left-brain hemispheres talk to each other and they experience a calming response.[46])
- ✧ A newborn that cannot wiggle into dangerous positions in their crib (like getting a leg stuck between the mattress and the railing).
- ✧ A reduction in the risk your baby will roll onto their stomach.
- ✧ Less waking due to startling (less arm flailing).

### ALTERNATIVES TO SWADDLING

Occasionally, a baby just doesn't like being swaddled.

Don't force it; it's not a requirement. First, you can try a modified swaddle, in which you place their hands on their chest instead of down by their sides, or a "half swaddle," in which your baby's arms remain outside of the tightly wrapped blanket.

If that doesn't work, you can double down on the other soothing options to help your baby fall asleep, like rocking them, walking them, breastfeeding, and/or babywearing (carrying them close to your body with a sling, small carrier, or wrap).

## Side Holding

Some babies find side holding soothing, particularly if they have reflux or other tummy troubles. You can hold them gently on their side in your arms or on your lap.

While you can use side holding to soothe your baby *before* sleep, remember that there is a difference between holding a baby on their side and putting them to sleep on their side. Side holding is wonderful; side sleeping is dangerous as they could easily roll onto their face or tummy, where their breathing could become obstructed, and get stuck there, particularly if they are swaddled.

> Babies should sleep on their backs to reduce the risk of SIDS, but not all of them like it. It's not a position they experienced in utero, and it may trigger their Moro reflex. To ward off that falling sensation that can trigger the Moro reflex, it may help if you hold your baby at a little bit of an angle as you put them down in their crib or other safe surface, so their feet are a bit lower than their head and their feet touch first.

## Shushing and White Noise

Often a gentle, rhythmic *sh-sh-sh* noise will calm your infant by reminding them of the mother's heartbeat in utero. You can also use a sound machine to help replicate the heartbeat.

A white noise machine can help you provide a sustained shushing. Dr. Karp suggests starting with an initial 100 dB to calm your baby and then turning it down to 65 dB. He also says that babies don't become dependent on it, and that you don't need to wean your baby from it until 3 or 4 years of age.[47] As an added benefit, white noise can also drown out other noises that might either keep your baby from falling asleep or startle them awake.

## Swinging

Gently rocking and swinging our babies to calm them is so instinctive that I scarcely have to mention it. The gentle motion soothes them by triggering a calming effect in the brain.

This simple, soothing motion can be incredibly powerful, but you may have to do a little experimenting to find what works for your baby. When I worked with 2-week-old Nicole, her parents found that she liked the swinging motion, but not in a swing—she preferred being in a carrier. (Her parents also found that while this worked well for soothing her in the first month, as she moved into month 2, she preferred swaddling, and that became their "go-to" soothing tool for her.)

It's fine to let your baby nap in a swing (if you have checked the safety of the swing with AAP recommendations) during the first 2 months. Please be cautious, however; swings have a scoop shape that can cause baby's head to fall forward toward their chest and block their airway. Always supervise swing naps and reposition their head in an upright position as needed.

For current swing recommendations, please see my products recommendations page at SleepLady.com/Products.

## Sucking

Sucking is a natural part of baby's self-soothing, so for parents who are worried that pacifiers are bad or the start of a hard-to-quit habit, take solace. Babies *need* to suck, especially during the first few weeks. It's not just about food; sucking itself is actually calming to the baby's nervous system. Babies who aren't offered pacifiers often suck on their fingers or their hands instead.

### CONSIDERING USING A PACIFIER?

Pacifiers are commonly used to help babies sleep. And for good reason! They can be a very effective tool.

If nursing, the AAP suggests waiting to use a pacifier until breastfeeding is well established (until your baby is latching easily and feeding well), but then recommends them for both daytime and nighttime sleep because they may protect babies against SIDS.

When considering using a pacifier, know that:

- ✡ It is a personal choice.
- ✡ Pacifiers don't help particularly gassy babies because they tend to swallow more air as they suck.
- ✡ If breastfeeding, you'll want to confirm that your baby is latching well and that a pacifier isn't impeding the process.
- ✡ You may find that a pacifier is helpful only in particular circumstances (for example, only at night, or only during the afternoon when extra soothing is needed, or just at the doctor's office).
- ✡ We suggest not keeping a pacifier in your baby's mouth the majority of the time, to allow them to communicate with you through vocalization.

If your baby spits out the pacifier, don't automatically re-plug it! You may be hampering their early attempts to communicate and interfering with your ability to differentiate between their cries. Sometimes they will want the pacifier back—and they'll let you know! But if you don't assume it's the pacifier they want, you may realize that they are trying to tell you something else.

## Additional Soothing Ideas

Sometimes just looking at your baby and talking to them is helpful. Their down-stairs brain is looking for you to attend to them, and just knowing that you are there and available to them can calm them down.

We've recommended rocking your baby, but sometimes just the obvious step of picking them up and holding them up on your shoulder can help soothe them. Again, part of what they are looking for is a response from you.

Moving your baby's body can also sometimes soothe them, as well. You can try:

- ✩ Rolling them on their side (only when they are awake, of course!).
- ✩ Folding their arms and legs in toward their chest (a fetal position might make them feel more like they are back in the womb).
- ✩ Gently placing your hand on their chest or tummy.

You can also try special "baby holds" that they may find soothing. Pediatrician Gabriela Zepeda recommends what is commonly called the "football" hold, where you lay your baby out on your arm on their stomach with their head turned to the side, their cheek on your palm, and their legs on either side of your arm. Another suggestion is the "baby bundle."[48] Here, your baby faces outward with their back to your stomach. You support their bottom with one hand and use your other hand to support their chin with your thumb and pointer finger.

## *Learn Your Baby's Soothing Cues*

Crying is an obvious cue that your baby is upset and needs soothing. But as you start to observe them, you will see that they let you know their needs in other ways, as well.

Your baby has two main cues as to their state of regulation that they will give you during this time.[49]

The first, which your baby might begin presenting toward the end of this month, is a relaxed open face with a smile and wide eyes. This lets you know they are comfortable and want to be engaged with you.

The second is looking away from you with glazed eyes or a frown or arching away from you with a stiff body. This means they have had enough or would like something different.

When your baby is upset, they are unable to move themselves or even understand why they don't like a particular situation. They can't limit their own stimulation. So this second cue may be their way of telling you that they would like you to do it for them. Thankfully, the caregiver brain is particularly wired to tune in to and recognize these cues. This is your chance to SOAR and determine if they are overstimulated.

Some additional cues you may notice when your baby needs soothing or calming:[50]

- A "cry face" or a frown.
- Excessive squirming or arching their back.
- Bracing their legs against you or their crib.

## Dunstan Baby Language's Burping Cue

A baby who needs to burp won't feel soothed and ready to fall asleep. How will you know if your baby needs to burp? They may seem uncomfortable after eating or pull their legs up toward their stomach. Or Dunstan Baby Language has a helpful "word" you can learn: "eh," which is the sound of your baby trying (but failing) to burp.[51]

If you hear this sound immediately after feeding, you can use the familiar over-the-shoulder burping hold with a repeated up and down rub to the back so your baby doesn't spit up what they just took in.

## Soothing Challenges

There are several soothing challenges that you might encounter this month.

## Soothing Colic

According to the Mayo Clinic, colic is "frequent, prolonged, and intense crying or fussiness in a healthy infant."[52] Pediatric nurse practitioner and PhD Maryanne Tranter shares that it appears in babies under 5 months with no known cause, and often occurs in the evening or toward the end of the day, which can set you up for difficulty getting your baby down for the night. If your baby has colic, it can be *very* frustrating to try to soothe them because they appear to be fussy for no clear reason.

While colic peaks at 6 weeks, Dr. Gaby suggests that we learn about colic at this age because up to 20 percent of babies suffer from it, and it can start as early as 2 to 4 weeks.

To be clear, all babies start to use crying as a form of communication at the end of their first month—this is expected, as you learned in the Development section. When we talk about a baby who has colic, we are referring to a baby who cries significantly more than other babies and has no obvious illness or other cause for crying.

### TREATABLE CAUSES OF COLIC

While some people might say you just have to "ride out" colic, the experts I've worked with find that it sometimes has specific treatable causes.

Dr. Maryanne shares that, like a fever, colic is a symptom, caused by something else going on with your child. She has found that colic can actually be the symptom of three different conditions:

1.  *Tongue and lip ties.* A tongue and/or lip tie (where the tissue between the tongue and floor of the mouth or the lip and gum is short or tight) affects latching and as a result baby can take a lot of air into their system while feeding, causing an uncomfortable stomach. Their difficulty feeding can also leave them frustrated and hungry.
2.  *Reflux (particularly silent reflux).* The discomfort associated with reflux, or when a baby's stomach muscle pushes the breastmilk or formula they drink back up, is major cause of crying that is often misdiagnosed as colic. You can tell when your baby is suffering from reflux because they'll arch their back rigidly in pain.
3.  *Food allergies or intolerances.* Soy and cow's milk are the most common because of an inability to break down larger proteins.

If you feel like your baby is particularly upset and crying excessively, you'll want to check with your pediatrician to make sure that none of these conditions are present, and if they are, address them. Your doctor may also look at other reasons for your baby's crying and discomfort.

## What Can You Do about Colic?

Holistic pediatrician Elisa Song reminds us that not all fussiness is abnormal and needs to be treated. The "colicky" period typically starts around 2 weeks of age and peaks at around 6 to 8 weeks of age, just as babies' brains are starting to mature, better equipping them to manage sensory overload. They're starting to smile and coo and engage with the world in a calmer, happier way. Your fussy baby may just need you to hold them, sit with them calmly, and know that they'll be okay.

However, when she sees a baby with colic in her practice, Dr. Song first takes a closer look at potential root causes. One potential root cause that she explores is food sensitivities. Particularly fussy babies may be reacting to something in the breastmilk or formula they're drinking. For formula-fed babies, a trial on a partially hydrolyzed or hypoallergenic formula may be beneficial. For breastfed babies, eliminating the most inflammatory foods from Mom's diet (dairy, gluten, soy, eggs, and corn) can do wonders to calm a colicky baby. She suggests that breastfeeding moms focus not on what they're missing, but on all the amazing foods they *can* eat, and

## Pediatric Acupuncture for Babies

As a pediatric acupuncturist, Robin Ray Green treats many common newborn conditions such as failure to thrive, reflux, colic, poor sleep, and teething pain. Gentle and effective non-needle techniques such as laser acupuncture used on the baby's meridian points can provide powerful help with soothing and sleep challenges.

For more details on pediatric acupuncture, please see Robin's website at RobinRayGreen.com.

nourish their body and their baby with delicious fruits and vegetables, wild and grass-fed meats and seafood, nuts and seeds, and gluten-free grains.

Dr. Song shares that holistic therapies can also be an amazing tool to help calm fussy babies. One study found that giving babies a combination of chamomile, ginger, lemon balm, and fennel significantly relieved colic symptoms. Some of these ingredients are found in Gripe Water, which many parents find helpful for their fussy babies. Giving a baby specially formulated infant probiotics that contain *Lactobacillus reuteri* has also been found to reduce colicky symptoms. Combination homeopathy medicines like Boiron's Colic Relief may provide quick, gentle relief as needed.

## Acupressure for Colic

Dr. Song has a special trick she teaches her parents with colicky babies. While nursing or bottle feeding, you can gently put pressure on and massage the CB12 acupuncture point, which is found at the midway point between the bottom of the sternum and the belly button (where the rib cage meets in the middle of your baby's chest). You can even use a drop of gentle essential oil like lavender or chamomile on the skin there; both scents are calming, and lavender in particular is known to relieve discomfort and physical pain.

When I started working with 6-week-old Jayden, his parents hadn't slept in days. It felt to them as if he cried *all of the time*! They admitted that they had been comparing Jayden to their neighbor's baby, who seemed delightful in the evening (and supposedly already slept for a five-hour stretch at the beginning of the night). It's hard to avoid comparisons, but I gently suggested to Jayden's parents that, in this case, it would make us all even more frustrated. They agreed!

Because Jayden seemed to need constant soothing, the family had no clear structure to their day. I understood how they'd gotten to that place, but I knew that a structure could help. We started by regulating Jayden's wake-up time so that his morning could start with a predictable routine. They were then able to add in a few more predictable routines throughout his day.

I then suggested they experiment with a few different soothing techniques—but only in the morning, when he was likely to be less fussy, so that they could get an accurate read on what worked to soothe him. They could then have these soothing tools in their pocket to try in the afternoon and evening when Jayden, like most colicky babies, got even fussier. They also followed my "3 PM Rule" (see box), which means that they reduced *all* stimulation every day after 3 PM.

Pretty quickly, they learned that Jayden liked white noise and a pacifier (thank goodness!). And eventually, the predictability of routines throughout the day also kept him calmer and easier to soothe. He wasn't quite as ramped up by the afternoon and evening.

---

### My 3 PM Rule

Within the 3 PM to 7 PM time period, I suggest:

- Turning off the TV.
- Dimming the lights.
- Soothing your baby with rocking and sucking.
- Bringing your baby into a separate calming room—either temporarily, or for the full period, if needed.
- Having a gentle "coming home" routine for other members of the family.

---

While Jayden's colic symptoms didn't disappear completely, these changes to the day helped to soothe both Jayden and his parents. He was less dysregulated at the end of the day and easier to soothe to sleep in the evening. Within a month, his fussiness was a distant memory, and Jayden's parents were happy to report that he was even ready for some gentle sleep shaping.

A lot of families that go through colic come out feeling a bit traumatized. This is totally understandable; it's a stressful time for both the parents and the child. No matter how endless it may seem, colic—thankfully—disappears eventually. I always encourage my families to do whatever works to soothe their babies through it.

## Soothing Eczema

Some babies suffer from eczema, which is dry, itchy patches on the skin. Eczema, especially if severe, can be very disruptive to sleep due to the discomfort it causes.

Holistic pediatrician Ana-Maria Temple, who has studied various causes of eczema, found a strong connection between eczema and the health of a breastfeeding mother's gut microbiome. She recommends that a breastfeeding mother log her food for a week. Often she'll suggest that the mother eliminate cow's milk, gluten, soy, and eggs to see if that helps the baby's eczema.

Your pediatrician can help you rule out an allergy to something transmitted through the breastmilk or in their formula, and recommend soothing lotions and topical treatments as well.

## Understanding and Handling Overstimulation

As mentioned in this month's Development section, your baby may start exhibiting extra fussiness between 3 and 12 weeks. This fussiness may appear particularly toward the end of the day.

According to renowned pediatrician T. Berry Brazelton's book *Touchpoints: Birth to Three*, a baby's immature nervous system gets overloaded as it attempts to take in and process stimuli throughout the day, and to compensate, baby "blows off steam in the form of an active, fussy period."[53] This fussiness allows the baby to effectively regulate themselves in a way that will last for another 24 hours.[54] As Dr. Brazelton says, it's like clockwork!

What can you do to help?

Limit the stimulation, including handling by others, that your baby gets throughout the day and particularly as the afternoon approaches.[55] Try following my 3 PM Rule (see page 89).

Preventing overstimulation makes your newborn easier to soothe, and a soothed, calm baby is easier to put to sleep. Limiting stimulation also keeps your baby from habituating. We want your baby to actually nap and wake rested rather than come out of a habituated state cranky and in need of more sleep.

 # TEMPERAMENT

Every baby is different, and some babies' temperaments—the way they take in, process, and react to their internal and external world—are more sensitive to stimulation than others. Their reactions may be stronger, and it can take longer to soothe them back to a calm state.

In my years as a sleep coach (and a mother), I've seen again and again how much a child's temperament can impact their sleep. How a child learns to sleep, what self-soothing techniques they choose, how adept they are at transitioning smoothly between sleep–wake cycles, and how they learn to self-regulate directly relates to their temperament. By learning about your baby's temperament, you'll get clues as to how to best soothe them and prepare them for sleep.

## Early Markers of Temperament

Some elements of temperament can be observed at birth, though because so many developmental events happen in the first 3 months, temperament is not fully evident until a few months later.[56]

Not all babies who are unsettled at birth or have a difficult beginning end up being what I call an alert baby (one who is keenly aware of their surroundings, active, intense, and highly sensitive both to internal and external stimuli), so temperament is not completely locked in at birth.

That said, many parents tell me that they saw clear indications of their baby's temperament as early as month 1. When I took my younger daughter, Gretchen, to the doctor during her first month, she squirmed excessively on the exam table (and almost rolled over!). The doctor said, "Oh! You have a Tigger." She explained that she had seen this temperament (which reminded her of Winnie-the-Pooh's bouncy tiger friend) before, even at this young an age. Sure enough, my younger daughter turned out to be an alert, sensitive, active child.

## Temperament and the States of Arousal

Your baby's temperament affects how they interact with the world. As your baby matures, you'll get used to how they respond to various situations. Your baby will also express their unique temperament as they move from being asleep to awake, and from fussiness to being content.

Dr. Brazelton identifies the six "states of arousal" that babies cycle through during the day:

- ☆ Quiet sleep state (non-REM).
- ☆ Active sleep state (REM).
- ☆ Intermediate state (transition between states).
- ☆ Wide-awake state.
- ☆ Fussy state.
- ☆ Crying state.

According to Dr. Brazelton, the way your baby moves from state to state will help you understand their particular temperament. An active and intense baby will move in and out of these states quickly. A laid-back baby will move more slowly.

Once you understand your newborn's particular cues and temperament, you can help them move gently through and between these states.[57] Learning who your baby is will help you know how to soothe and respond to them.

## Alert Babies

For alert babies, it is harder to shut out the world, especially when they are trying to go to sleep. These babies are particularly sensitive. Some have a low tolerance for stimulation and are overly sensitive to environmental disruptions. These babies may have difficulty coping in loud, intrusive, or overwhelming situations.

I told you about my "Tigger" baby squirming on the pediatrician's exam table. Even the nurses in the maternity ward the month before noticed her temperament. When she joined our family, I had to switch gears because this baby was clearly not like my first. I had heard that a second baby was supposed to be more adaptable and "would go with the flow" since they came into the world with a sibling. Not this one! I had to pivot . . . and quickly. What worked for her sister wasn't going to work for this one. I had to watch her closely and log whenever I saw patterns and cues. I made mistakes along the way, of course. But she helped me become a better mother—and a better Sleep Lady—as time went on.

Most of the babies and children I sleep coach are alert. Their filters are open wider to the world than those of other children, and they (and their parents) need a little extra help as they learn to sleep. Eventually, with our help, they learn to create their own filters, but until then, *we* are their filter.

## Supporting Your Baby's Temperament

You'll soothe and prepare your baby for sleep differently according to their particular temperament. You'll also care for them differently when they wake in the night.

### Read Your Baby's Cues

Spending a lot of time engaging with your baby is how you will learn their cues and respond to them quickly, but you don't want them to get overstimulated from too much interaction. They are not used to all of the environmental input around them, and they may not understand what they feel inside their own bodies. They can't tell you exactly what is making them uncomfortable. (Luckily, as they mature, they will get better at showing you what they need. I remember feeling so relieved when Carleigh told me for the first time that she had an earache! I didn't have to guess what was bothering her.)

Perhaps you realize toward the end of this month that every time your baby fusses and you try to feed them, they don't eat well. They only eat well when they're already soothed. This is a big "aha" for your SOAR process. You can check "feeding" off the list as the way to soothe them—even if they're hungry.

Experiment. Be your baby's detective. You are both learning how to "speak" to each other. By appropriately responding to your baby's cries now, you also help them transition to "non-crying communication" in the near term—between 12 and 16 weeks.

## Supporting Your Alert Baby

Parents of alert babies need to be even more responsive to their baby's cues. Gentle Sleep Coach Macall Gordon, MA, reminds us that an alert baby's reactions don't just show you what they would *like* but also speak to their actual *needs*. It's important that they be allowed to express these needs and that you react to keep their stress hormones balanced.

Sleep can be particularly challenging for alert babies, so give them extra soothing and know that the process of getting them to sleep (and later, teaching them to fall sleep on their own) might take longer and require you to go slower.

My daughter Gretchen was particularly sensitive to stimulation, cried a lot, developed eczema, and besides having reflux, only fed well when in a quiet, dark setting. Now, this is not to say that my first child was an angel baby—she did her fair share of crying and had feeding problems, as you heard at the beginning of this chapter—but she was more adaptable and less outwardly intense. I share this with you to remind you that our task is to figure out who we have been given and then learn to understand, read, and respond appropriately to them as an individual.

### Tips for Alert Newborns

- It can be harder to read the sleepy cues of a highly alert baby, which I believe is because they are so engaged in the world that they don't show those cues as clearly and often not until overtired. They might not rub their eyes, for example, but their eyes might appear glassy instead. And signs that they are sleepy might not appear until you have gotten into your pre-bed sleep routine (which is why it's helpful to have a sense of when your baby usually gets tired and start the routine to lead up to this time).
- Alert newborns may be easier to soothe (and feed) in a separate room away from the excitement of the rest of the family.
- Gentle massage works very well for these newborns, while anything remotely stimulating might be more intense for them at bedtime.

- You may find that your alert baby does not sleep on the go. Or you might find they can in the first month or so but not later. Respect that need, and work with them—you can't "train" them to sleep in bright light and noise, nor should you. It's like suggesting that a natural "night owl" can easily become a "morning person" or a coffee drinker must switch to tea (and also like it). You may need to arrange your schedule to allow them to take their naps at home, in a consistent location (or at least in the dark and with quiet).
- Co-sleeping might not work for your alert newborn because their alertness and curiosity will keep everyone up at night. These babies are particularly sensitive to movement, touch, and smell.

The most important thing to understand when caring for your alert baby is that some of the suggestions I make throughout this book won't work immediately for your little one. You're in a more challenging situation than the parents down the block whose baby starts sleeping through the night easily at 3 or 4 months. Your job will be a little bit tougher. And with that, it's also important to know that you are not doing anything wrong.

In the coming chapters we'll help you better understand what makes your alert baby special so that you can effectively apply the tips we share with you. And don't despair, even alert babies learn to sleep! I know this professionally as well as personally. It may take a tad longer and you may have to use a more gentle, sensitive touch, but it will happen!

## *Look at Your Expectations*

Pediatrician Shoshana Bennett shares that as you get to know your baby, you may find that your baby's temperament isn't what you expected. (There may be a lot about the experience of parenthood that is not what you expected!) She says that some parents even put this difference on themselves and feel that they have made a mistake. She reminds us that a baby's temperament is something that they are born with and that all we can do is accept and love them. Accepting your baby's temperament will allow you to better soothe your baby in a way that truly works for them.

#  GETTING YOU AND YOUR BABY TO SLEEP

Sleep is why you've joined me on this journey following your baby over their first 5 months, and now that we've set the foundation with Feeding, Attachment, Soothing, and Temperament, we can talk about your baby's sleep at this age and other ways to support it.

It takes a lot of energy for babies to be awake, take in their new surroundings, and grow both physically and cognitively. Sleep is how they restore themselves. When your baby sleeps, you can also sleep—letting you restore yourself, too.

We want your baby to eventually fall asleep on their own, but at this stage, your job is to help them as they learn the process. Luckily, sleep itself is what helps their brain solidify their daily learning!

## What to Expect

As always, I'd like you to understand what your baby is currently experiencing so you know what they are capable of and how to help them meet their needs.

During the first 6 to 8 weeks, your baby's sleep cycle is unorganized. This means that they do not fall asleep or wake up at predictable times.

Your baby's sleep will develop in a specific order:

- ✫ Night sleep develops around 8 weeks.
- ✫ The morning nap begins to develop around 12 weeks.
- ✫ The afternoon nap begins to develop around 16 weeks.

These developments all occur "around" a certain time, but there is never an exact date. I have found that the naps often develop even later than these averages, so don't despair if you get to 16 weeks and find your baby still doesn't nap well, even in the morning.

So long as your baby's sleep-wake cycle remains underdeveloped, try not to have great expectations about them sleeping long stretches. And don't worry about creating "bad habits." Your baby needs you to soothe them to and back to sleep right now, however you can. It's very common for parents to try a number of different ways to soothe their babies during this stage.

## Sleep Needs in Healthy Full-Term Babies

There are wide ranges of time given for how much an infant should sleep within a 24-hour period, but the most important finding in infant sleep research in the last 15 years is that **sleep needs can vary by 8 or 9 hours in a 24-hour period in babies 6 months and under**.

> Generally, newborns up to 3 months old sleep for **14 to 17 hours during each 24-hour period**. This includes both daytime naps and nighttime sleep. Most newborns can be awake for only 1 hour at a time (or 1½ hours maximum) before becoming overtired.

As you can see, this range is very broad, which is why it is important to not compare your baby to your neighbor's, friend's, or sister's—two babies' sleep needs can vary by a very large amount. There is no typical newborn schedule or normal sleep average for babies under 6 months.

Your goal is to help your newborn get restorative sleep within this healthy range. My goal is to give you tips and tricks to help you do this. But it is essential to have realistic expectations. During this time, your baby will sleep in short spurts around the clock. They will need to feed often throughout both the day and night. At this stage, there is not much predictability to sleep patterns or lengths.

## Sleep States

The sleep states your baby passes through now are similar to the ones they experienced while in utero. In the first 3 months of life, their sleep will evenly cycle between active or REM sleep and deep or non-REM sleep.

### Active Sleep (REM Sleep)

In the first 20 to 30 minutes of sleep, your infant is in an active state of sleep. This phase is sometimes referred to as "light" sleep and consists of REM (rapid eye movement) sleep.

In active sleep, your baby is processing and mentally storing all their experiences from the day, which plays a critical role in brain development. Blood is flowing to your baby's brain, bringing nutrients to active brain cells.

You will be able to observe rapid eye movement under your baby's closed eyelids when they are in this state; their nervous system is active as well. Other characteristics your infant will display in active sleep are:

- ✡ Irregular breathing.
- ✡ Facial expressions (grimacing, puckering of lips, opening/closing mouth, and/or frowning).
- ✡ Sucking and other body movements (twitching, startling, stretching).
- ✡ Vocalization (whimpering, crying out, whining, grunting), particularly at night.
- ✡ Easily startling or awakening.

---

### Easily Awakened during Active Sleep

Does your baby wake as soon as you lay them down? It is very common for young babies to wake easily during the 20 to 30 minutes before they transition into deeper sleep. Try waiting until your newborn's body and eyes are still to put them down. When they are in a deep sleep, they are more likely to stay asleep when they are laid down.[58]

---

### DEEP SLEEP (NON-REM SLEEP)

After active sleep, your infant will move to deep sleep, also sometimes called "quiet" sleep. Again, this stage lasts about 20 to 30 minutes.

During deep sleep, your baby is very still, with eyes closed, rhythmic breaths, and very little muscle movement. Many new parents check frequently during this phase to make sure their baby is breathing! Quiet sleep is restorative, allowing the brain to rest.

Characteristics of deep sleep:

✼   Closed eyes with no rapid eye movement.

✼   Regular, shallow breathing.

✼   A still, quiet body.

✼   No spontaneous movement (though your baby may startle, they will remain asleep).

In a deep sleep, your baby may be able to selectively tune out sounds and bright lights and is difficult to awaken. Try not to wake or interact with them at this time.

## Supporting Your Baby's Sleep

I don't recommend sleep coaching at this stage. Even something as simple as putting your baby down to sleep drowsy but awake, a common sleep coaching step, is not recommended at this age. A recent study found that starting the drowsy-but-awake

---

### Understanding Sleep Crutches

You may have heard someone refer to their baby having a *sleep crutch*—a term I use in my book for children 6 months to 6 years old. A sleep crutch is what I refer to as a *negative sleep association*—anything that has to be done *to* or *for* a baby to put them to sleep and back to sleep that they can't do independently, such as nursing to sleep, rocking to sleep, re-plugging their pacifier (which they won't be able to do themselves until 6 months at the earliest), or a combination of several of these!

At this age, almost all babies have at least one sleep crutch. It's expected, because they have not yet learned how to fall asleep on their own. Maybe you rock them to sleep with white noise on in the background, or perhaps they cannot fall asleep without their pacifier. I will show you ways to gently wean your baby off these crutches in a few months, once the time is right for you both.

practice at 3 weeks had no effect on the baby's sleep once they reached 6 months of age.[59] Your baby may be able to naturally put themselves to sleep if they are a bit drowsy, but don't worry if they aren't able to. It's perfectly natural for them to need your help at this point, and again, you are not creating any bad habits.

You'll learn more about my gentle Baby-Led Sleep Coaching in future months. However, I do have sleep *shaping* steps you can take now to improve your baby's sleep!

## Avoid Day-Night Confusion

Avoiding day-night confusion will be a major focus of this first month. This is the place where your help can make a difference in your baby's sleep and set a solid foundation going forward.

Many babies are born with their days and nights mixed up. This means they are prone to sleeping during the day and might be more wakeful at night. New babies sleep when they are tired, wake for a feed or some connection, then go right back to sleep.

Remember that your baby is operating from their primitive brain. At this point, their internal clock is not yet developed. Until a baby develops their circadian rhythm (the hormonal cues that tell them when to be asleep and when to be awake), they don't have a good sense of whether it is daytime or nighttime. Circadian rhythms don't become fully mature until about 6 months (though the beginnings of these rhythms can be seen around 3 months).[60]

In the meantime, it's your job to help them know when to be asleep and when to be awake. Here are some actions you can take to help your baby start to distinguish between night and day:

- ✯ Make sure that your baby is eating regularly throughout the day. (You may even decide to wake your sleeping baby for a feeding during the day—not letting them sleep longer than 3 hours.)
- ✯ Expose your baby to bright outdoor light during the day (or if this isn't possible, open the shades and turn on the lights inside).
- ✯ Keep your baby in a low blue light or dark and quiet environment at night.
- ✯ Keep nighttime activities in dim light and focused on feeding and diaper changing rather than playing.

Your bedtime routine is also helpful for signaling that nighttime is approaching. Eventually, dimming the lights and slowing down the activity around them will give their brain the message that it's time to slow down. Their brain will then secrete the hormone melatonin that will make them drowsy (this starts happening in the third or fourth month).

## Fill the Daytime Nap Tank

At this age, the key to making sure that your baby gets enough sleep within each 24-hour period is to ensure they get an appropriate amount of sleep during the day. I call this **filling your baby's daytime sleep tank**. And I suggest you fill your baby's daytime sleep tank any way you can: by holding or safely lying with your baby, and/or by feeding them to sleep and then back to sleep when they need it. Contrary to popular belief, the better your baby sleeps during the day, the better they will also sleep at night. When they become overtired, their body secretes cortisol, which wakes them up further. As a result, they can end up waking more frequently at night as well as earlier in the morning before they are truly rested.

## Create a Consistent Bedtime Routine

Toward the end of this month, when you feel more confident about caring and feeding for your baby, is a great time to create a consistent bedtime routine. At this point, your baby might take a short nap while you and your partner have dinner. You might then bathe them and give them a short, relaxing infant massage, and then begin their bedtime routine. A bedtime routine can be as simple as dimming the lights at the same time every night and then nursing, bottle feeding, or rocking your baby to sleep in the same location while listening to the same song.

Initially, for the first several months, this routine may happen at *your* bedtime. But as you start seeing a pattern in your baby's cycle of waking, feeding, and sleeping, keep an eye out for a time that starts to make sense as *their* bedtime (a time when they consistently get drowsy or, perhaps, after which they tend to get particularly fussy and difficult to soothe). During month 2, you'll start to ever-so-slightly regulate their bedtime so that it comes at approximately the same time each evening, within a 30-minute window. If it doesn't start moving earlier naturally by month 3, we will guide you through how to move it forward gently over the course of a few nights. Having a familiar bedtime routine will help make this process easier, by clearly signaling to your baby that bedtime is coming, even if it is a bit earlier than they are used to.

Naps also benefit from a pre-sleep routine, which will often be shorter and just involve feeding or rocking. In this first month, many babies can nap in a bassinet in the living area of your house or next to your bed when you decide to also take a daytime nap. It's still important to quiet the environment and dim the lights for naps, but it's not as important as it is at bedtime and during nighttime feedings. It helps to act as if their internal clock is already developed (even though it is not). We all sleep better on a regular schedule and in a quiet, dark, cool environment.

The good news is that during this month and maybe until month 3 or 4 (depending on your baby's temperament), your baby may be fairly portable and flexible in their daytime sleep—able to sleep on the go or in a swing in the living room. Enjoy this flexibility while it is here! The more alert your baby, the sooner it will end.

## Regulate the Wake-Up

Also toward the end of this month, you may notice your baby is beginning to wake around the same time each morning. Look for a pattern. Perhaps they usually feed at 5 AM and 7:30 AM, but don't easily drift back to sleep after their 7:30 AM feeding. You'll then know that their wake time for the day is around 7:30 AM. Take this as their cue to start the day—even though you know that their first nap will start shortly.

If you do not yet see a pattern, that's okay! It will come—perhaps in a few weeks. If your log notes that your baby's wake time remains particularly inconsistent, for example 7 AM one day and 9 AM the next, you may decide to simply pick a time to start the day and try that out consistently for a week or so. A regular start time will help start to organize your baby's naps during the day, which will then help you determine when to start their bedtime routine in the evening.

## Create a Sleep-Friendly Environment

It is important to create a sleep-inducing environment for your newborn, particularly for night sleep. For more detailed suggestions, please see page 34.

Your baby's sleep environment is important. We shouldn't be trying to "teach" babies how to sleep in noise or bright light, especially as the result may be habituation rather than restful sleep. Rather, we should be creating an environment that supports sleep. Your baby's temperament is also a factor; as you've learned, some babies are naturally more sensitive to their environment than others.

---

### ☁ Sleep Lady Tip ☁

Swaddling, white noise, and a dimly lit environment will help your baby sleep easier.

---

## Learn the Sleepy Cues

Your newborn will not have a regular sleep schedule at this time, so you'll want to put them to sleep whenever they seem drowsy. Your newborn will give you cues that say *I'm getting sleepy*, and it's very helpful to learn to recognize these cues. In addition to generally becoming quieter, your baby may show some of the following:

- ☆ Decreased activity.
- ☆ Slower motions.
- ☆ Weaker or slower sucking while feeding.
- ☆ Lack of interest in their surroundings.
- ☆ A less-focused gaze.
- ☆ Drooping eyelids.
- ☆ Irregular breathing.
- ☆ Yawning. (To avoid a meltdown, try to put them down after the first yawn!)

A crying baby can be a sign that you have missed their sleep cues and they have become overtired. If this is the case, they'll be tougher to soothe to sleep, which is why we encourage you to get out your magnifying glass and see if they are trying to communicate their drowsiness to you in some other way before the crying starts.

Drowsiness serves as a transition both into and out of sleep. If left alone, your baby may go to sleep or they may instead gradually awaken. If they have been up for a while (more than 1 hour) when you start to see these cues, this would be a good time to put them down to sleep.

## Dunstan Baby Language's Sleepy Cue

According to Dunstan Baby Language, your baby will make a vocal "owh" sound when they are becoming tired, due to the yawning reflex.[61] The "owh" sound can be heard both pre-cry and with a full cry. The trick is to catch the "word" before it is accompanied by crying so that the baby is easier to soothe and calm enough to put to sleep.

# THE ELEMENTS OF BABY-LED SLEEP SHAPING (MONTH 1)

**(1) CREATE A SLEEP-FRIENDLY ENVIRONMENT**
- Room-darkening shades.
- Soothing colors.
- White noise.

**(2) CREATE DAILY ROUTINES**
- At bedtime, use your consistent, soothing routine. Do this in your baby's nursery if you plan to eventually transition them there, even if you are currently room sharing.
- Create a shorter pre-nap version of your pre-bed routine.

**(3) PREVENT OVERSTIMULATION (FOLLOW THE 3 PM RULE)**

**(4) DON'T LET YOUR BABY SLEEP THROUGH A DAYTIME FEEDING (OVER 3 HOURS)**
- Have your baby's last nap end 1 to 1½ hours before their bedtime.

## Co-Sleeping This Month

Some parents do not intend to co-sleep but change their mind once baby arrives and find that co-sleeping works best for them. If this is you, please take a look back at Before Birth, where I share a number of thoughts on co-sleeping, to learn about the importance of creating a safe co-sleeping space.

If you had initially chosen to co-sleep, now that your baby is here you can see if it is working—whether it is too stimulating for your baby or too disruptive for you. Co-sleeping has to work for the whole family, and now you can actually test the sleep plan you created for yourselves.

## Sleep Challenges at This Age

It may seem that everything involving sleep is a challenge at this age. Fear not! Things will get easier. In the meantime, there are some aspects of your baby's sleep that might be more of a challenge than they need to be.

### Recognizing When Your Baby Is Habituating

After I'd become The Sleep Lady, I was at a friend's party—just a small casual barbecue—and a couple had brought their newborn. These new parents kept handing the baby off to each other to try to calm him while chatting with guests in the loud, brightly lit kitchen. They each tried rocking, shushing, feeding, and soothing him, and finally came over to me to ask if I had suggestions.

By this time, I had learned about habituation. I looked around at the environment he was in and had a strong feeling that he was overstimulated and trying desperately to tune out, shut down, and habituate without great success. I suggested that the parents carry their baby into a quiet, dimly lit room in another part of the house and try calming him there.

It was like magic. We were all silent as they held him, and after a few minutes, he quieted and then opened his eyes. I explained that a baby this age doesn't have the ability to say, "It's too much." Their only options are crying or habituating. And habituation was difficult for this little guy when he was being jostled in a space that was loud and brightly lit.

The new family had enjoyed their time at the party but decided to pack up and head home—knowing that when their baby was older, it would be easier for him to handle more stimulation and to communicate his needs even more clearly.

If they had stayed, they would have been repeatedly subjecting him to what, for a newborn, are high levels of stimulation. He would have likely habituated, appearing to have gone to sleep, but then slept poorly that night. It wouldn't have been worth it!

Habituation is short-lived and begins to wane slowly after 8 weeks. By 2 to 3 months of age, few infants can still shut down, and almost none can shut off completely.

Still, it's valuable to learn to recognize the signs of habituation, however short-lived, because, if it happens regularly over a few days, it can lead to fussy feedings and shorter naps. A baby who is regularly practicing habituation may seem jittery or anxious when awake and can explode into lots of crying. They will often wake crying and find it difficult to settle down even after feeding.

Keep your eye out for the warning signals that lead to habituation and learn what overstimulates your baby. It is not the same for all babies. Some babies have a low tolerance for stimulation and are even more sensitive to environmental disruptions. This temperament will make them even more susceptible to habituation.

Experiment with darker, quiet areas to see if that helps protect your baby's sleep cycles and results in more prolonged stretches of sleep.

### How to Recognize Habituation in Your Baby

☆ Pulling in their arms and legs and closing their eyes.

☆ What looks like deep sleep in brightly lit and loud surroundings.

### How to Prevent or Recover from Habituation

☆ Move to a dim, quiet location.

☆ Soothe your baby before trying to put them back to sleep.

☆ Make calming your baby's environment and filling their daytime sleep tank your priority the following day. This may mean staying home and having a day of quiet and relaxation for everyone.

## PREMATURE BIRTH

If your baby is born before their projected due date, you will be working with your pediatrician to attend to any particular needs your baby might have. Perhaps unsurprisingly, when it comes to premature babies there are a few important differences in how we approach sleep.

## Adjusted Age

You will probably hear your pediatrician mention your baby's "adjusted age." This age is based on their projected due date, and can seem a bit silly within the first several months since your newborn is clearly not "zero" or "younger than zero." But knowing your baby's adjusted age will help you understand their development, as your baby's development will follow their adjusted age rather than their age based on their birth date. **The expectations you can have for your newborn's sleep will also be in line with their adjusted age. Your baby's readiness for sleep shaping and coaching will also match their adjusted age.**

## Sensory Processing

Lindsey Biel, OTR/L, pediatric occupational therapist and coauthor of *Raising a Sensory Smart Child*, shares that our senses are how we comprehend the world. We see, hear, and touch things. We experience gravity, and we use our bodies to move. Once received, all of this sensory input—both from the environment and from inside our bodies—is then integrated in our central nervous system in a neurological process referred to as *sensory processing*. Sensory processing is what enables us to feel, think, and behave in proportion to what's happening inside and around us, and it's something we become more efficient at as we grow.

Lindsey says that children born prematurely are at increased risk for sensory-based difficulties. A preemie with sensory issues can experience being rocked as frightening. Changes in head position may feel like the world has turned upside down. The sound of a lullaby may be painful to the ears, and a flickering fluorescent light may look like lightning flashes. What seems normal to us can easily overwhelm a child with sensory issues, and this is especially true for preemies whose brains and bodies are not yet able to handle the barrage of sensory input from the world.

In part because of this difference in sensory processing, premature babies frequently have shorter daytime and nighttime sleep and decreased quality of sleep in the first 2 years.[62] It helps to understand your preemie's development so you can respond to them accordingly.

## *Lindsey's Tips for Helping Premature Newborns Sleep Better*

- ✬ Reduce overwhelming visual stimulation (an "interesting" mobile may not be the best idea!).
- ✬ Keep your baby swaddled for a good part of the day, but always make sure their hands are free, so they can suck on their fingers and fists when they are developmentally ready. Ensure they have opportunities each day to kick and stretch their little legs, too.
- ✬ When holding your baby, tuck in their arms and legs so that they are in a secure, flexed position, as they would be in the womb.
- ✬ Keep them warm, with a household temperature of 68 to 72 degrees and extra layers. In general, a warmer temperature is preferable for premature babies who often have challenges with thermoregulation.

Feeling overwhelmed? One of our Gentle Sleep Coaches would love to help you create your sleep shaping plan and support you through the process! Visit FindaSleepCoach.com.

## YOUR SELF-CARE

Now that your little one is here, you may understand why we were putting so much emphasis on committing to self-care. Like many parents or caregivers of newborns, you are probably exhausted. Not only that, but there is a lot more going on as well.

## *Parent Brain Development*

Yes—"baby brain" is a real thing! It's not just that new parents think that they are going crazy. Birth parents and adoptive parents (and, in fact, all caregivers!) exhibit brain changes as they care for babies.

Dr. Oscar Serrallach, an expert in the field of postnatal health, writes in *The Postnatal Depletion Cure* that birth mothers temporarily lose the ability to multitask, become hyper-focused, and develop a higher sensitivity around sight and touch.[63] Their brains instinctively slow down to help them focus on their baby's subtle cues and communications.

When someone becomes a parent, major structural and functional changes occur in their brain that make them more effective at caring for an infant.[64] *All* caregivers experience brain changes, regardless of whether or not they carried and gave birth to the child, and in cultures where there's more communal caregiving, this is even more the case. Researchers speculate that these brain modifications are an evolutionary adaption that has supported the success of humans over many thousands of years. If an infant's birth mother were to die, the baby would need another caregiver or caregiver network to be able to step in.

Nannies and childcare workers also experience these brain changes, though the extent of this change depends on the amount of time they spend caring for babies.[65] Just think! Your little one is getting a community of caregivers specially adapted to care for them. It takes a village, and the village's brains change, too.

As your baby's parent or caregiver, be gentle with yourself as you find yourself becoming more sensitive and single-focused. For birth mothers, these changes can last up to 2 years.[66] While disconcerting, they are beneficial for helping you recognize and meet your baby's needs.

## Preventing Postpartum Depletion

As a birth mother, the "postpartum depletion" that goes along with your brain changes can be a particular challenge. That's why we focus on how you can support yourself so that you can be of even more support to your baby.

You learned a little bit about postpartum depletion in the previous chapter. It is a group of symptoms affecting all aspects of life that can stem from physiological issues, hormone changes, and the disruption of the normal circadian rhythm.[67] While all caregivers may experience some elements of postpartum depletion—experiencing exhaustion due to sleep deprivation, and often feeling socially isolated as they care for their baby in the first few months—birth mothers, and especially nursing mothers, have the additional challenge of having provided or still providing needed nutrients to their babies.[68]

In other words, the exhaustion you're feeling can be caused not only by a lack of sleep but also by postpartum depletion.

> Mothers who have just given birth are physically healing, and that is a challenge in and of itself. If you have just given birth, make sure that you are working with your doctor to get the support that you need for the healing process.

To head off postpartum depletion, Dr. Serrallach suggests:

- Getting good sleep when you can.
- Eating healthy foods.
- Taking restorative supplements.
- Drinking lots of water.
- Being active each week (he recommends both a restorative yoga class and taking walks).

Dr. Serrallach also suggests taking a social media vacation to give yourself a break from comparing yourself to other parents, and your baby to other babies. He shares, too, that this is not a time to entertain visitors, who should instead be given tasks to do when they stop by to meet the new baby.[69] Dr. Serrallach urges parents to "play first and work later,"[70] which sounds a lot like Radha Agrawal's Joy Practice (see page 47).

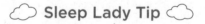

## Sleep Lady Tip

Limit visitors to close family. Become a short-term hermit.

## Baby Blues versus Perinatal Mood and Anxiety Disorders (PMADs)

Baby blues—that is, brief episodes of mild mood changes—are extremely common the first few weeks after giving birth. You may feel moments of sadness or experience mood swings; you may cry; and you may feel vulnerable, stressed, or anxious. **But baby blues are transient. They go away in about 2 weeks.** Dr. Shosh shares that if feelings of intense sadness, anxiety, or mood swings last longer than this, you may be experiencing PMADs.

PMADs have biological components. In birth mothers, pregnancy hormones plummet, affecting brain chemistry, and a history of depression is a risk factor. But exhaustion, stress, and new-parent anxiety also play a role.

Under the PMAD umbrella are six specific disorders: postpartum bipolar disorder, postpartum panic disorder, postpartum obsessive compulsive disorder, postpartum psychosis, postpartum post-traumatic stress disorder, and the most familiar, postpartum depression.

I see forms of PMAD in a lot of the families who come to me for sleep help. Exhaustion is a risk factor for depression, and depression makes it harder to sleep shape successfully, which in turn breeds more exhaustion.

If sad feelings or anxiety are overwhelming, if you experience any thoughts of harming yourself or your baby, or if your symptoms start to interfere with your daily life, get evaluated for postpartum depression immediately.

It's also important for the people close to new parents to be on the lookout for symptoms of PMADs. Parents experiencing postpartum depression don't always recognize the signs or may already be too depressed to take action.

According to psychologist Dr. Shosh, postpartum depression is the most common PMAD; globally, about 15 percent of women who give birth experience it. This condition can also appear in fathers[71] and adoptive parents.[72] Traditionally, it was thought to begin in the first month after birth, but now we know it can also occur later in that first year. Letting it go untreated is not good for the parent, and it's also not good for the baby, who may have more trouble forming a secure bond with a parent who is depressed, emotionally flat, unresponsive, or anxious.

Developing a PMAD does not mean you are a bad parent or an unloving or failed one. It does not mean that you will not feel better and enjoy parenthood for many years to come. It does not even mean you will experience a similar depression after every birth (although you are at higher risk).

Dr. Shosh finds that there are a few risk factors that make certain people more susceptible to PMADs, but no one is immune. It can affect anyone regardless of education, strength of character, culture, personality, or background. Many women develop symptoms during pregnancy, but for others, the onset happens after delivery. Some of the most common symptoms include difficulty sleeping at night when the baby is sleeping, change in appetite (usually a decrease), anger, high anxiety, despair, overwhelm, and low self-esteem.

Many people don't realize they're suffering from depression because the symptom bothering them is anxiety—not a stereotypical sad, numb, or lethargic feeling. An anxious mom might be fully dressed with makeup on and very productive during her day. Postpartum anxiety sometimes includes obsessing about one's own or the baby's health, which leads to behaviors such as making extra doctor appointments and repeatedly checking the baby's breathing at night.

It's important to remember that you don't have to be a birth mother or primary caregiver to develop a PMAD. Studies show that while a baby's primary caregiver (irrespective of gender or biological relatedness) will experience more hormonal changes than secondary caregivers, all caregivers can experience physical and mood changes. And remember, it's not just internal changes that impact PMADs; the external stress of sleep deprivation and other changes to your life and routine can contribute, too.

PMADs are completely treatable when the right help is provided. If you or your partner are experiencing signs of a PMAD, please contact your doctor and check out Postpartum Support International (Postpartum.net). To download Dr. Shosh's Wellness Plan, with suggested supplements and steps you can take to prevent PMADs, please see DrShosh.com/WellnessPlan.

## Your Sleep and Well-Being

One of the best pieces of sleep advice I can give new parents is one you've probably heard before: Sleep when your baby sleeps. I know that might seem difficult right now, but I suggest making it a priority.

At this stage, it is ideal to get 5 hours of sleep in one stretch each night (for nursing mothers, this is once breastfeeding has been established). This uninterrupted sleep will help protect against PMADs. If you have already been diagnosed with a PMAD, this sleep is even more important.

If you need help to get this block of sleep, ask for it. Split nighttime duties (with your partner or another caregiver) so that you are not completely exhausted by the time the sun rises. Make sure, also, that you are open to accepting help when it is available or offered.

We've spent a lot of time talking about creating the right sleep environment for your baby, but it's worth looking at yours, too. If you have only a precious few hours to rest, spend them in an environment that supports deep, restorative sleep.

---

### ☁ Sleep Lady Tip ☁

Your baby's sleep is very inconsistent during this time; they will sleep and feed around the clock. Plan for this by napping when you can and at least getting some rest whenever baby goes down.

---

## Calming Yourself Calms Your Newborn

In *Calm Mama, Happy Baby*, Derek O'Neill and Jennifer Waldburger write, "As a mom, you've probably noticed by now that when you're calm, you feel connected to your baby and your instincts, and it's easier to make clear decisions about your baby's needs. When you're stressed, on the other hand, you feel disconnected from yourself and from your baby, too, and things can feel a lot more chaotic and confusing."[73] Connection with your baby is particularly important at this stage.

To help keep your baby regulated, it's helpful to keep an eye on your own stress level, and manage it so that *you* can stay regulated (or get yourself back to a regulated state). O'Neill and Waldburger remind us that we can actively take ourselves out of a fight-flight-freeze and remain nonreactive in the face of our babies' fussiness.[74] We can practice doing this through meditation, a Joy Practice, yoga, and/or breathing exercises—which is why we offer some specific breathing and mindfulness practices in this book.

Dr. Serrallach suggests trying the "four in/seven out" breathing technique,[75] which cardiologist Mimi Guarneri uses to calm her highly stressed cardiac patients: breathing in evenly for a count of four and breathing out evenly for a count of seven. This is a lovely calming practice that you can do even while holding your baby or trying to get to sleep at night.

The way we respond to our baby impacts them both in the moment and in the future—because it influences the development currently occurring in their brain. Just remember that when your baby cries and your efforts to soothe them aren't

---

## Acupuncture for Those Who Have Just Given Birth

Pediatric acupuncture specialist Robin Green shares that acupuncture can help reduce and eliminate pain from the trauma of childbirth, including neck, shoulder, back, sciatic, and breast pain. Most importantly, acupuncture helps treat postpartum depletion by balancing the nervous system and activating the body's self-healing mechanisms, thereby helping new mothers with fatigue, difficulty sleeping, and postpartum depression. It can also play an important role in promoting lactation for mothers with insufficient breastmilk, which is common with postpartum depletion. Dr. Serrallach says, "I've seen regular acupuncture sessions cut a new mum's depletion-recovery time from the typical 6 to 9 months down to 3 months."[76]

working, it's not your fault. I know that it can be hard not to take it personally, but staying calm will help you to take a step back and SOAR with your newborn.

## HOLD TIGHT!

What an amazing and challenging time your baby's first month is!

I know that you are doing your best to navigate it, and you are succeeding. While it may feel like you are fumbling through your days and nights, that just means you are learning. And so is your little one.

Things will change before you know it. Soon your baby will be ready for more sleep shaping. In the meantime, here is what I suggest you focus on during month 1 of your baby's precious new life.

## ONE-PAGE FAST TO SLEEP SUMMARY

**Month 1 Theme:** *Your baby is operating from their primitive brain. You, as a parent, have experienced brain changes that let you better care for your baby.*

### What to Focus on This Month

1. Accept help and offload anything that isn't focusing on your healing and your newborn.
2. Learn about and avoid habituation (page 105).
3. Implement the 3 PM Rule (page 89).
4. Aim for one feeding your baby a minimum of 8 times in 24 hours.
5. Help your newborn overcome their day-night confusion (page 100).
6. Try for 1- to 5-minute tummy time sessions (page 59), two to three times per day.
7. Establish a daily feeding and sleep routine (not schedule).
8. Create a sleep-friendly environment (page 34).
9. Create pre-sleep routines for bedtime and nap time (page 101).
10. Don't let your baby sleep through a daytime feeding (over 3 hours).
11. Commit to at least one self-care activity a day . . . something just for you!

### What Not to Worry About

Sleep training! You *cannot* create any bad habits at this age.

For a printable PDF of this month's FAST to Sleep Summary plus helpful book bonuses, go to SleepLady.com/NewbornSleepGuide.

# Your Baby's Second Month

## *4 to 8 Weeks*

*This month, we'll share some gentle, soothing tools for both your baby and you. We'll address your baby's increased fussiness and look at how to soothe colic, allergies, and eczema. We'll talk about a few nighttime and nap strategies as well.*

### Parent Spotlight: Emily

*Mother of a 7-week-old son, Ryan, who was born full-term and healthy*

I was exhausted and questioning my ability to be a good mother . . . even to the point where I thought perhaps a nanny would do a better job. Ryan hated being swaddled and hated his bassinet even more.

I was nursing him six to eight times a night in hopes of trying to comfort him before his crying escalated so much that it would take what felt like hours to settle him down. We didn't have any kind of schedule, and it seemed like bedtime was anywhere from 8 PM to midnight—which, of course, meant his morning waking time was different each day. There was definitely no nap schedule. I consider myself an "attachment parent," and I was terrified that letting my baby cry it out would emotionally damage him. At the same time, I was desperate for sleep. I had read about other babies his age and weight sleeping through the night after parents let them cry it out. I was prepared to stop breastfeeding altogether since that seemed like the only solution.

I learned from Kim that at Ryan's age, he doesn't fully know the difference between daytime and nighttime and hasn't organized his sleep and feeding patterns. She explained that I wasn't "ruining" Ryan by feeding him at night and that he was neither developmentally nor physically ready to night wean at this young age. I was so relieved! She also told me that I didn't need to stop breastfeeding to improve his sleep—that there was huge variability in babies under 6 months, and it wasn't fair to compare Ryan to the other 2-month-olds I read about on social media.

Kim encouraged me to keep a sleep log and not let Ryan sleep through a feeding time during the day. I started to wake Ryan for the day at 8 AM and moved toward a consistent earlier bedtime . . . all without crying or sleep training. I learned that I needed to be his "external clock."

What a game changer! I no longer felt anxious in the morning about what the day would hold. Now we had a rhythm to our day, and I wasn't racked with guilt over spoiling him or fears that I was creating lifelong horrible sleep habits.

Kim taught me how long Ryan could be awake at this age before getting overtired. I got so much better at reading his cues—for sleep, hunger, and discomfort. We didn't start nap training (which he wasn't ready for) but instead focused on getting him great daytime nap sleep (even if it meant I had to wear him in a carrier). I added white noise and watched how long he was awake, and before I knew it, he didn't mind the swaddle!

When Ryan and I were ready, Kim said we could try putting him down at bedtime with the *Jiggle and Soothe*. [You'll learn this method in this chapter and maybe even try it toward the end of the month.]

All of these changes, however small, ended with us all being on a more consistent schedule and giving us a nice flow to the day. I got better at reading Ryan's cues, and I felt more hopeful about my role as a mother. And soon, his night sleep improved. He still woke for a few feedings, which was appropriate, but it wasn't every hour or two. It all felt more doable! I also reminded myself that this was going to get better, so I could enjoy spending time with him and my new role as a mother.

## MORE PREDICTABLE RHYTHMS AND ROUTINES

At this age, your baby's sleeping and feeding patterns will start to become more predictable. The time between feedings will start to spread out, and at around 6 to 8 weeks, you will begin to see one longer stretch of sleep during the beginning part of the night.

As we learned last month, routines are an important part of your baby's life. Babies truly "live in the moment," so having a rhythm and pattern to their day gives them an inkling of what comes next. Building familiar and consistent routines around your baby's days and nights will help them feel safe and secure. They keep them from feeling like they are living in a whole new world each day. And falling into more predictable patterns will eventually help with sleep (yay!), because they will be easier to soothe and the routines will cue them when sleep is "up next." Not to mention, routine will also help you as a parent. All ages like the comfort of routines!

The good news is that you've probably settled into some gentle routines without even realizing it! You may sing the same song before naps or when your baby is fussy, or perhaps you always tickle your baby's feet after a diaper change.

These little acts amount to a much bigger picture for your newborn. Remember that the world is a lot to take in and can be very overwhelming to your baby's still very fragile nervous system.

> Some routines you established in the first month may not be as effective as your baby heads into the second month because of all the changes your baby is going through. As always, paying attention to your baby's cues will help you best support them through their growth.

Flexibility is tremendously important right now. This is not the time to get caught up in rigid schedules, nor to follow the clock down to the minute. Simply create a nice, consistent flow to your day. Do things in the same order on a regular basis. Observe your baby's patterns to figure out what their natural flow is and blend your routines in. Your routines may feel repetitive, but, to be frank, that is how you know you're setting them up well.

For routine suggestions, please see Month 1.

## Routines Help the Whole Family

One of my Gentle Sleep Coaches worked with a 7-week-old whose family schedule was all over the place. The baby's bedtime and wake-up time changed each day, and she was awake and fussy from 11 AM to 3 PM. Not surprisingly, the parents spent hours throughout the day trying to get her to nap.

After looking at a week of their log and asking targeted questions, we suggested a consistent yet flexible framework for their day. The parents started by waking her at the same time each morning to create a regular start to the morning. They then noticed when she typically fell asleep in the evening for a longish stretch and made that her bedtime. We shortened the time she was awake between naps. The parents also reduced the baby's stimulation after 3 PM because we found that they were inadvertently overstimulating her by trying to do "more" to put her to sleep.

Your routines don't have to include *everything*. Massage (more on that in Soothing), bath, song, story, tummy time, and feeding may be too much before bed. I suggest picking two or three elements (such as dimming the lights, feeding, swaddling, and/or singing) to set the stage for sleep and tell your baby that they are safe and loved. You'll find a routine that fits your family's needs.

## DEVELOPMENT

As your baby begins to reach new developmental milestones, you'll notice that there is a period of "disorganization" that occurs right before a burst in development.[77] Just when you've settled into a groove or set of routines that works for your little one (progress!), you find they're suddenly fussy at an hour when days before they had been consistently calm. You may think to yourself, *What's wrong with my baby? Are they sick? Not getting enough to eat?* Rest assured, this is all normal.

## Brain Development

Your baby is still operating from their downstairs brain, slowly moving to using their emotional brain (see page 54), but this development takes time. They won't start using their emotional brain—which allows them to learn rudimentary ways to soothe themselves—until between 4 and 6 months. But the transition has started.

Their downstairs brain still needs to know that their feeding needs are going to be met and that they are safe. This is still your job. And we're here to help you! This month builds on what you learned last month by putting the focus on reducing stimulation and soothing your newborn by learning to read their cues and following the SOAR process.

## The Sensations Leap

According to researchers Hetty van de Rijt and Frans Plooij's book *The Wonder Weeks,* which outlines the developmental milestones to expect in babies' first 2 years, around week 5, your baby enters into a new world of "sensations." At this stage, they are able to better see and hear their surroundings.[78] These new senses can be exciting but also potentially overwhelming.

In conjunction with (or just before) this developmental change (which *The Wonder Weeks* refers to as a "leap"), your baby may exhibit a fussy period, particularly demonstrating what van de Rijt and Plooij call the "three Cs": They are "cranky, clingy, and crying."[79] You can help your baby by providing the closeness they crave and also by helping them explore their new world by providing opportunities to use their heightened senses.

I'm sorry to say that during this period, your little one's sleep habits might suffer. Crying can become excessive (more on that shortly). So, it is particularly important to create a calming environment in the afternoon and early evening. We will help you soothe your baby through this leap.

## PURPLE Crying

Your baby's rapid development during their first few months of life can cause them stress, which is why you may be seeing crying increase, sometimes to excess. Pediatrician Dr. Ronald Barr, in partnership with the National Center on Shaken Baby Syndrome (NCSBS), developed the term "the Period of PURPLE Crying" to describe this completely normal stage of infant development, which starts around two weeks of age, peaks during the second month, and decreases by month five. The NCSBS partners with hospitals and early intervention programs to educate parents that this crying period is a normal part of development.

The PURPLE acronym highlights the identifying characteristics of this period as a reminder to parents:

P: Peak of crying
U: Unexpected
R: Resists soothing
P: Pain-like face
L: Long-lasting
E: Evening

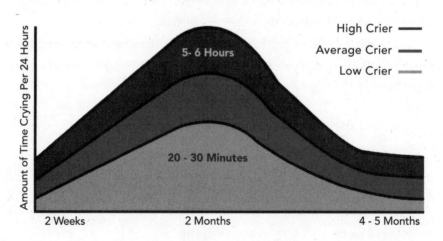

## Curves of Early Infant Crying
### 2 Weeks to 4 - 5 Months

Dr. Barr and the NCSBS wants parents to know that although this stage can be stressful, it is a phase your little one will move through. With this knowledge and the ability to prepare for the possibility of heightened crying, parents will be better equipped to calm themselves as they calm their babies.

The Period of PURPLE Crying is not the same as colic. As pediatric nurse practitioner Dr. Maryanne Tranter explains, "Colic is a diagnosis. PURPLE is a list used to describe characteristics of crying in this age group."

Because we know that this age is the beginning of increased crying, this chapter will continue our focus on helping you read your baby's cues as well as share pointers on soothing your baby (and you!).

## Supporting Development for Better Sleep

As in your baby's first month, there is one activity in particular you can engage in with them that will help support their development and establish a strong foundation for self-soothing and better sleep: tummy time.

### Tummy Time

Tummy time is still an important part of your baby's day—one that can be rolled (pun intended) into a routine. As you learned in Month 1, positioning your baby on their stomach will help them strengthen their neck and arm muscles, which will help them roll over in the future (and let them soothe themselves by doing so, rather than having to rely on you to help them change positions).

In month 2, your baby can handle **up to 20 or 30 minutes of tummy time a day, broken into several sessions**. Pick times when your baby is alert, aware, and social (but not right after feeding, so they are less likely to spit up).

 FEEDING

By this time, you will have started to find a good feeding pattern, and feeding itself will have become more efficient, requiring less time. Your baby has regained their birth weight. It's helpful to address any outstanding feeding issues at this time.

## Feeding at This Age

In the second month, babies usually take **2½ to 4 ounces per feeding every 2 to 4 hours**, whether breastfeeding or bottle feeding. **You can expect your baby to still need feeding at night (the number of times will depend on your little one).** However, they may feed fewer than eight times within 24 hours if they are getting more at each feeding.

---

### Average Breastmilk or Formula Intake Calculations

The daily amount of breastmilk or formula your baby needs is:

body weight (in pounds) multiplied
by 2.2 = number of ounces

For example, if you have a 10-pound baby . . .

$10 \times 2.2 = 22$ ounces of milk or formula

Then, to figure out how much your baby should be getting each time they feed, divide this by the number of feedings.

So, a 10-pound baby eating 8 times a day should be having roughly 2.75 ounces of milk or formula per feeding.

Most babies will increase the amount of milk or formula they drink by an average of 1 ounce each month before leveling off at 7 to 8 ounces per feeding by 6 months.

---

If you have been keeping a feeding and sleep log, you may see a daily pattern emerging with one longer stretch of sleep between feedings at night. Your baby may then go longer between feedings in the morning and want to feed more frequently toward the late afternoon and evening. Keep this new pattern in mind as you tweak their afternoon and bedtime routines.

I don't recommend forcing a schedule—particularly if your baby is experiencing feeding challenges. However, you might be seeing something like the following if your baby is eating every 3 hours with some cluster feedings in the later afternoon and early evening. (Because your baby's nap schedule may still vary greatly, we've left out nap times and lengths.)

**7 AM:**  Feeding and diaper change (your baby will likely wake for the day around this time and be awake for only 45 minutes to 1 hour; their nap length will vary)
Nap

**10 AM:**  Feeding and diaper change
Nap

**1 PM:**  Feeding and diaper change
Nap

**4 PM:**  Feeding and diaper change
Nap (either here or after the next feeding)

**6 PM:**  Feeding and diaper change

**9 PM:**  Feeding and diaper change (your baby may go to bed around this time)

**1 AM:**  Feeding and diaper change (this is after their one long nighttime stretch, which will eventually get longer)

**4 AM:**  Feeding and diaper change

## Feeding Challenges

Addressing eating and digestion challenges continues to be one of the most important things you can do to help support sleep. You'll want to work with your pediatrician and lactation consultant to identify and get help with any challenges you or your baby are experiencing. We have a few tips for those we see regularly.

### Latch Challenges

Making sure that your baby has a deep, strong latch is one of the best ways to support established breastfeeding. A poor latch can keep a baby from getting enough milk at each feeding, frustrate them (because they are either uncomfortable or hungry and craving a faster milk flow), and affect a nursing mother's milk supply. If a baby ends up particularly fussy due to a poor latch, they can be difficult to calm and soothe before sleep and they may wake earlier due to hunger.

Gentle Sleep Coach Heather Irvine, CLEC, shares, "I met Sarah when her daughter was 7 weeks old. She was struggling with her baby's frequent wakings." Sarah said that her daughter was very restless at night and would only sleep for short periods of time.

"As a lactation professional," says Heather, "I was able to assess Mom and baby and found that the baby was struggling with her latch." Heather went over some breastfeeding positions with Sarah and demonstrated some feeding tips. Pretty soon, the baby began to have more efficient feeds, and over the course of the next few nights, this helped lead to longer stretches of sleep with fewer wakings. When the baby did wake, she was easier to feed and settle back to sleep because she easily latched on quickly, ate more efficiently, and didn't get overly upset like she used to, struggling to feed.

## Reflux versus GERD

There's spit-up . . . and then there's spit-up!

As you learned in Month 1, gastroesophageal reflux disease (GERD) occurs when the valve between the esophagus and the stomach regularly allows contents of the stomach to flow back up into the esophagus and mouth. It is less common than regular spit-up, and unlike regular spit-up, which doesn't affect sleep, can seriously disrupt your baby's rest and happiness.

Be aware that reflux doesn't always present the same way. When my daughter Gretchen was 2 to 3 weeks old, she developed feeding challenges. While nursing, she would pull off and arch her back, but she wasn't spitting up excessively. She was also hiccupping regularly post-feedings and crying a lot. By the time she was 8 weeks old, I was at my wit's end as to how to get her to feed comfortably, the way she had in her first several weeks of life. When I took Gretchen to the pediatrician, the visit was about to conclude with no helpful advice on the subject when I took a break to feed her. As usual, she pulled off and arched her back, and the pediatrician realized immediately that she had *silent reflux,* meaning she had the pain and surges of acid without the spitting up.

If you suspect that your baby may have GERD, check with your pediatrician. I have noticed that babies with GERD, much like alert babies, can be very sensitive to their environment and remain so even after they are no longer suffering from

GERD. They react more to stimuli such as bright lights, crowds, food, and textures. Pay attention to their sensitivities post-GERD just as you would a baby with a sensitive temperament, and be mindful of their environment, from potentially itchy clothing to possible food triggers in breastmilk or formula ingredients that might upset their tummy.

> Dr. Anthony Loizides, a pediatric gastroenterologist, shares that as long as your baby is awake and with a caregiver, the best position for easing their reflux is lying on their left side. This position is not recommended at night, however, in case baby accidentally rolls onto their belly.

## Cluster Feeding

*Cluster feeding* refers to when baby-led feeding sessions bunch closer together at certain times of the day. In your baby's first month, you may have found yourself feeding them in multiple back-to-back sessions because they hadn't yet started settling into a feeding pattern. As a natural feeding pattern begins to emerge this month, these "clusters" of feeding sessions will start to stand out. Cluster feeding is normal and natural at this age, but it can feel frustrating to new parents because it may seem that the baby is fussy and eating all the time.

You may also hear cluster feeding referred to as a *marathon feed*. In some cases, it may feel like your baby is eating practically nonstop for 2 to 3 hours at a time.

Cluster feeding can occur at any time of day but usually happens in the afternoon or evening and often matches up with a baby's fussiest time of day. And it's often, but not always, followed by a longer sleep period. It's as if your baby is filling their tank ahead of time. You may find that they eat every hour from 6 to 10 PM and then do a six-hour stretch of sleep immediately after, which at this stage is considered "sleeping through the night." Cluster feeding can be a good sign that your baby is ready to sleep for longer stretches. Check with your pediatrician to confirm whether or not you need to wake your baby to feed them during long stretches at night.

During cluster feeding, your baby may appear fussy. You may see a cycle in which they cry and pull off the breast or bottle for a minute or two and then begin to feed again. Your baby might want to remain near or on the breast or bottle for this period of time. Cluster feeding can coincide with a late afternoon fussy period, but to be clear, they aren't just trying to self-soothe; they are pushing for more nutrition.

If you see a pattern of cluster feeding emerging, keep your schedule open during this time of day. For example, if your baby has started cluster feeding between 4 and 7 PM, don't plan to go to the grocery store at 5!

### CLUSTER FEEDING, BREASTFEEDING, AND MILK SUPPLY

When a baby nurses for a few minutes and then pulls off, fussy and crying, and then nurses for a few more minutes and then pulls off, it often leads parents to wonder if their milk supply is okay. Generally, the milk supply is fine; baby just happens to be engaging in cluster feeding during a normally fussy time of day.

As a breastfeeding mother, the more often you empty your breasts, the higher the fat content of the milk. The longer you go without feeding, the more water your breastmilk contains—there might be more milk, but that milk contains less fat.

Sometimes milk flow is slower in the evening, which can frustrate babies, and might lead to the pulling-off-the-breast behavior. Again, this does not necessarily mean there's a milk supply issue.

If you notice a pattern to your baby's cluster feeding, as a nursing mother you can prepare for it by staying particularly hydrated during this time of day.

 ## ATTACHMENT

A secure attachment is crucial to your child's future ability to interact with others, develop empathy, and self-regulate, and the key to forging a secure attachment is caregiver responsiveness. Attachment happens as you and your baby develop your own unique language and your baby learns to trust that you will help them meet their needs.

Gentle Sleep Coach Macall Gordon, MA, shares that our babies learn self-soothing by experiencing brief moments of distress, like learning to roll, having their diaper changed, and feeling hunger before they are fed, alongside a caregiver they trust. With your help, they experience how to go from a dysregulated state to a regulated one. Once they learn what a regulated state feels like, they learn to ask for your assistance to get there. Eventually, they learn to get there on their own through physical actions like looking away, rolling to their side, or sucking their thumb. But at this stage, they are not yet capable of these physical actions and therefore still need your help to soothe themselves out of a distressed state.

In their book *The Calm Baby Method*, pediatric occupational therapist Patti Ideran and pediatric gastroenterologist Mark Fishbein share that your baby may start exhibiting clear attachment behaviors as soon as 6 to 8 weeks old. For example, they can start to show a slight preference for one of their caregivers (nursing babies often prefer their mother because of the combination of comfort and relief from hunger that comes with her presence).[80] Their most important mission at this age is learning to give signals that will get others to respond to their needs.[81]

With the increased crying this month, you (and all of your baby's caregivers) will be responding more and experimenting. Remember, it's okay to get it wrong! You and your baby are learning about each other. The important thing is just that you respond.

Consistently comforting your baby now lays the foundation for them to become confident and secure on their own in the future, which can help with sleep coaching in a few months. Don't worry about spoiling your baby in these early months. Our ultimate goal is independence, and focusing on responding and being attentive now is what will get us there.

##  SOOTHING

You may be at a point when you thought you were getting a handle on your baby's cues and how to soothe them, only to hit this increased fussy period and find that your best tricks no longer work, or that what works one day doesn't work the next. Continue to experiment! This section on soothing offers more ideas you can try.

As you reach the end of this month, habituation wanes, but your baby hasn't yet mastered self-soothing. They are still practicing. Your job is to work with what they have available to them skills-wise and keep your expectations realistic. This month it's key to be prepared to soothe late-afternoon fussiness and take advantage of your baby's developing senses in trying new calming tools to prepare for sleep.

If your baby has entered the Period of PURPLE Crying stage (see page 122), they may be upset for no particular reason and simply need soothing (more on how to do that shortly).

That said, at this age your baby might be trying to communicate something to you by crying. As you are trying to soothe them in preparation for sleep, deciphering the meaning of their cries can be particularly important.

When your baby cries, you can use the following list to interpret their needs.

### Common Causes of Crying

- ✫ Feeding issues:
  - Hunger. (How long has it been since their last feeding? Was it a good feed? Is this a cluster feeding time of day?)
  - Tongue tie.
  - Not getting enough milk when breast or bottle feeding due to low supply or slow milk flow.
  - Fast milk flow (bottle or breastfeeding).
  - Oversupply of milk (breastfeeding).
  - Upset tummy.
  - Allergy.
- ✫ Diaper needs changing.
- ✫ Discomfort. (Are they too hot? Too cold? Are their clothes scratchy?)
- ✫ Tiredness.
- ✫ Overstimulation. (How long have they been awake? Babies are more easily overstimulated when overtired. Have there been any changes to their environment in the last couple of days? Are they in a loud place like a restaurant, with siblings running around and new smells from the kitchen? Have they been handled too much by family?)
- ✫ Medical issues:
  - Illness.
  - GERD.
  - Constipation.

— Diaper rash.

— Eczema.

— Torticollis (when the neck muscles regularly contract, causing the head to twist or tilt to one side).

Each time your baby is fussy, it may be something different that calms them. Also, keep in mind that you may not always be able to calm them down—you may just need to wait for the crying to pass—but just being there for them, trying to help, and showing them love will make all the difference.

## *Tips for Soothing Your Baby*

> Don't Forget Dr. Karp's 5 S's:
>
> - Swaddling.
> - Side holding.
> - Shushing.
> - Swinging.
> - Sucking.
>
> Check out Month 1, page 79, for the specifics.

 Pacifiers This Month

Pacifiers are particularly popular this month because they:

☆ Allow your baby to soothe themselves during this period of general fussiness.

☆ Are a handy soothing tool for breastfeeding mothers, so that they don't have to be "on call" to soothe at all times.

☆ Can ease ear pressure during air travel.

As magical as pacifiers can feel, it's important to pay attention to your baby's cues so you understand when they need to feed as opposed to when they are just soothing themselves with sucking. Remember, the pacifier is just one tool in your soothing toolbox.

> Don't worry! Pacifier use as a baby won't affect your child's teeth and palate formation as a teen—this will be mostly based on genetics.[82]

## WHEN TO WEAN

If you choose to use a pacifier, you don't need to start weaning your child until they are approaching 15 to 18 months, when they are likely to get more attached. However, you may decide to limit use to nighttime sleep (or you may choose the opposite and use it only during naps) as your baby gets a little older.

Some parents have their baby suck on a pacifier until they are calm and then, once they are drowsy, remove it, so their baby falls asleep without having to suck. It might be worth a try!

## Soothing through Senses

As your baby's senses develop, they get temporarily fussier, and yet their heightened senses of touch, hearing, smell, and more will also help you soothe this fussiness, including in preparation for sleep. You can soothe through more than one sense at a time if you like.

## TOUCH

Body contact through touch activates opioids and oxytocin in the brain—which lower the stress levels in both you and your baby.[83] Touching and holding calms your baby, and it has the added benefit of bolstering your attachment to each other.

Ways to calm through touch:

- ✫ Rubbing your baby's palms or clapping their hands together.
- ✫ Rubbing your baby's feet from toe to heel.
- ✫ Gently exercising your baby's legs, waving their arms, or lifting them up and down.

☆ Breastfeeding (even if they have already fed, your baby will benefit from the body contact and may need nonnutritive soothing/sucking).

☆ Holding your baby while bottle feeding (versus propping up the bottle).

☆ Taking a warm bath or shower together.

☆ Concentrating on your breathing while holding your baby close (taking a deep cleansing breath from your diaphragm and exhaling slowly and completely).

## Infant Massage

Spending any relaxed, one-on-one time with your baby only brings positive results for both of you, psychologically and physiologically (and for your baby, developmentally). But the benefits of stopping and really connecting with your baby through infant massage are astounding.

A study done at the University of Warwick found that massage helped babies under 6 months sleep better, cry less, and be less stressed. Researchers found that levels of the stress hormone cortisol were lower in babies who were massaged.[84] Massage positively affects all body systems, from digestion and circulation to the brain, nervous, and immune systems. It can also help ease discomfort from gas, constipation, teething, and congestion.

Plus, infant massage gives you the opportunity to stop and really pay attention to your baby's cues and learn from them.

We recommend building some dedicated massage time into your routine to help you quiet and relax your little one. But be flexible and watch for signs from your baby that it is time to stop: crying, stiffening of limbs, or irritability. Your strokes should be firm and not ticklish. Research and try out some different techniques until you find the ones that they enjoy the most. Start when your baby is in a quiet and alert state, right after a feed, or another time when they are not sleepy.

## MOVEMENT

Movement often helps calm and settle babies—it's generally assumed that this is because it reminds babies of the sensations of being in the security of the womb. This is the idea behind swinging your baby to soothe them. You can use movement with your baby in a number of ways:

- Holding and rocking your baby (or swaying with your baby).
- Taking them for a walk in a stroller or baby carrier.
- Placing your baby in a baby swing or vibrating chair (while supervised).
- Sitting on an exercise ball and bouncing with them.
- Wearing your baby around the house in a sling or carrier, for example while dancing or putting away laundry.
- Dancing with your baby.

## DISTRACTION

Trying new activities and exploring new surroundings activate dopamine, a neurotransmitter that controls the pleasure center of the brain and regulates emotional responses. When you distract your baby with new experiences, you soothe them. You can try:

- Bringing them into a different room.
- Walking around the house or their room and pointing out various items.
- Stepping outside into the fresh air.
- Making silly faces at them.

## SOUNDS AND SMELLS

Sounds and smells can activate positive feelings and lower stress levels. Use them carefully, however, as they can also be overstimulating. You can try:

- Playing familiar music and singing along (combine this with movement by moving both of you to the rhythm!).
- Talking to them quietly and soothingly.
- Playing white noise, sounds of the womb (more of a "whooshing" sound than white noise), or heartbeats.

✧    Turning on the stove fan or bathroom fan.

✧    Introducing (in small doses) calming scents like lavender or vanilla.

When trying these soothing tools, first experiment with one at a time. And if one tool doesn't work, take a beat before jumping to a new one. Moving between activities too fast or in too jarring a way can upset your baby even more. Moving slowly between two soothing solutions will allow your baby to settle into the new approach and help you accurately gauge their response.

## Soothing Challenges

You may encounter two main hurdles to effectively soothing your baby this month. The first is colic, which we went into in depth in Month 1. The second is overstimulation, which we introduced in Month 1 (see page 86) but discuss in more detail here.

### Overstimulation

As a baby's senses become more developed, their brain and body have to start processing all of the new information that is coming their way. This incoming information stimulates both their brain and body. Overstimulation happens when they have taken in too much information (either all at once or over time, as overstimulation can build up over the course of the day), and it becomes too much for their brain and/or body to handle. An overstimulated baby is usually a fussy baby, and very difficult to soothe to sleep.

Along with reading your baby's cues, it helps to regularly take note of the level of stimulation in your baby's environment. Being aware of sources of stimulation lets you either reduce the stimulation or soothe your baby before they become overstimulated (and then fussy!). Unfortunately, trying to get your baby to adapt or get used to stimulation doesn't work—exposing them to loud noises during nap time does not help them "get used to it."

When I worked with Theo's family, his parents told me that they actively tried to give each of them the chance to bond with him every day. Theo's dad worked during the day and looked forward to coming home to give his son a bottle in the evening. He treasured this time! He would chat with Theo while feeding him in the brightly lit living room—sometimes with the TV on or some music playing. Eventually, Theo started regularly crying and had difficulty eating during what had previously been a pleasant time for the two of them. After looking at Theo's daily routines and temperament, his family and I determined that by the end of the day, Theo was overwhelmed from all of the daytime activity and was just looking for a quieter bonding session.

Theo's dad started using this early evening feeding time to give his baby his undivided attention by holding him but in silence. Theo no longer responded with cries and unfocused eating. And Theo's dad rescheduled their "chats" for the quiet mornings before he left for work.

## Habituation in Month 2

As you saw in the Development section of this chapter, although habituation wanes at the end of your baby's second month, they can still habituate up to that point. This makes it even more important to be aware of their environment and watch for over-stimulation so that you can recognize the difference between stressful habituation and true deep restorative sleep.

When Carleigh was 5 weeks old, her father and I attended a friend's Greek wedding. We were the first of our friends to have a baby, and we were excited to show her off (but not hand her off to everyone at the wedding). I brought her to a quiet room to feed her, and then when the band started, she "fell asleep." Everyone was amazed at how she was able to sleep through all the noise, and so were we.

She had been a reasonably good sleeper for her age up until that night, when she woke multiple times and was almost impossible to soothe. Even nursing didn't help. We were all a wreck the next day. I didn't learn about habituation until a few years later, at which point, I looked back and understood what she had been doing—and why, when she later woke in the quiet night, she cried and was inconsolable.

If you think that your baby may be habituating but aren't sure, pay particular attention over the next 24 hours to whether they seem rested. If not, examine their environment and activities to see if overstimulation might be preventing restful sleep.

## Overstimulation Cues

Your baby is looking for you to help them when they are overstimulated. Some cues for overstimulation include:[85]

- ✩ Blueness around the mouth, redness in the face, and/or mottling of the skin, such as blue crisscross lines (my younger, alert baby exhibited this cue, and I had originally been assured it was because she was cold!).
- ✩ Fast and erratic breathing.
- ✩ Sucking in a burst-pause pattern while eating (if not addressed, the next stage is sucking that is very fast, hard, and often noisy).
- ✩ Loss of normal head control.
- ✩ Increased startle response.
- ✩ Legs pulled up to the chest.
- ✩ Looking away and avoiding eye contact.

If you use the SOAR process to *Assess* what was happening before these cues appeared, you will likely find that some overstimulation occurred. By noting what it was for the future, you can help your little one from heading down the path to overload again.

When you see these cues, you'll want to respond quickly—before your baby moves to the next stage, intense crying.

## How to Hold Off a Meltdown

When I refer to a "meltdown" at this age, I mean uncontrollable red-faced and full-body crying that can be very challenging to soothe quickly.

If you are paying attention to your baby's environment and realize that they have experienced multiple forms of stimulation over the last few hours, you can hold off a potential meltdown by turning off the TV, if on, and turning on some soft jazz or spa-like music. Often, just taking your baby to a different, quieter room and dimming the lights will help.

You can also make plans to keep future meltdowns at bay by arranging to do any errands and outings in the early part of the day and then staying home, following my 3 PM Rule (see page 89). Better yet, delegate those errands to someone else!

 ## TEMPERAMENT

You'll see even more of your baby's temperament this month. It will appear in the way they react to you and objects around them, including the way they react to overstimulation (though keep in mind that the increased crying common toward the end of this month is not necessarily related to your baby's temperament).

### Alert Babies

You've heard a bit about my alert baby, Gretchen. Her pediatrician called her "my Tigger," and she was more aware of her surroundings than the average baby. She was more sensitive to bright lights and loud noises and more distracted during feedings. She was also more difficult to calm before sleep.

Child temperament expert Mary Sheedy Kurcinka, EdD, has her own name for the little ones I call alert babies. She calls them *spirited* babies (and later on *spirited* children).[86] Dr. Kurcinka shares a vast amount on these babies in her fantastic book *Raising Your Spirited Baby: A Breakthrough Guide to Thriving When Your Baby is More . . . Alert and Intense and Struggles to Sleep*. In addition to the traits that Gretchen displayed, Dr. Kurcinka says these babies can appear to have additional sensory sensitivities,[87] such as not liking large crowds, having their face washed, or wearing or being touched by certain fabrics or textures. They might not react well to a change in the schedule or environment and may also be more cautious than other babies in new environments. Their most noticeable trait, however, is their fussiness. On the fussiness scale, these babies often go from zero to one hundred in the blink of an eye. I've seen the same patterns in the alert babies I've worked with over the last 25 years.

Kurcinka writes that "20–25 percent of all babies born are spirited . . . genetically wired to be highly alert and intense."[88] She explains that these little ones have "highly reactive arousal systems," which makes them quick to ramp up and then slow to calm down again.[89] Kurcinka provides a helpful "zone system" for parents and other caregivers of spirited and alert babies to help identify where their baby is at the moment:[90]

- ✢ Green Zone: Everything is fine, and the baby's needs are being met.
- ✢ Yellow Zone: The baby is starting to struggle and needs a response.
- ✢ Red Zone: The baby's arousal system has been overloaded. They are distressed and in need of a massive response.

With alert babies, it's most important to catch them before they reach the red zone—particularly as you're heading toward bedtime or nap time, as they will be more difficult to soothe to sleep. Learning what cues they give in the yellow zone will help you know when it's time to step in with soothing.

It can also be helpful to monitor *yourself* in relation to these zones. Alert babies are particularly sensitive to the states of those around them. They may start to fuss if you are feeling stressed. Being aware of your own stress level means that you can pass your little one off to a partner if needed, or soothe both of you by putting them in a front carrier and dancing to soft, soothing music with them.

## How to Support Your Alert Baby

I've got some specific tips for caring for these little ones, who can seem completely different from those "easier" babies you've heard about:

- ✢ Feed them in a quiet room. Other babies might happily feed undistracted with the family bustling around them, but your alert baby may do better with just the two of you alone, separated from the noise.
- ✢ Respond to your alert baby quickly, because the time frame between "slightly fussy" and "completely melting down" is shorter than with other

babies. Be ready to SOAR, moving through the process quickly, and have soothing techniques at the ready for some of their common cues. (Parents of alert babies often carry around multiple pacifiers, and sometimes a front carrier stowed in the stroller basket in case their little one gets fussy and needs to be calmed down by being carried.)

✧ Set up your alert baby's sleep environment carefully, as it will affect them more than other babies. Your alert baby might be more affected by light during naps and do better with room-darkening shades, or perhaps you'll find that you need a dimmer night-light to keep them calm during night feedings.

✧ Plan to have baby home in time for their usual afternoon nap time. Many babies will sleep on the go up to 3 months—when they start to become more aware of their surroundings, making it more difficult to fall asleep, and their circadian rhythm develops, leading them to wake more completely between sleep cycles—but your alert baby might not be so flexible.

✧ Experiment with different types of touch (you can give them a massage or try kangaroo care—see page 77), but note that not all alert babies respond well to touch due to sensory sensitivity.

 ## GETTING YOU AND YOUR BABY TO SLEEP

At the beginning of this month, you are still your baby's external clock. During the next few weeks, however, their own circadian rhythm will start to emerge. You'll see it start to appear between 6 and 8 weeks, when you'll see one longer stretch of night sleep emerge—usually at the beginning of the night. The consistent and soothing routines we've encouraged you to put in place really pay off when you start seeing this longer stretch.

### What to Expect

Some parents are told to start sleep training at this age and to use the "cry it out" method to teach their baby to sleep. As you learned in Start Here, we disagree with this advice for a number of reasons. As a reminder, the "cry it out" method is not effective for babies (particularly at this age) because:

- ☆ They are still functioning from their downstairs brain and therefore cannot filter out overstimulation on their own.
- ☆ They are not mentally or physically capable of soothing themselves by sucking on their hands, turning their heads away from overstimulation, or finding other methods of comfort, and so they need you to soothe them.
- ☆ They can't learn when they are in a dysregulated state (overly upset and crying).

In addition, babies produce cortisol when they are distressed (when their needs aren't met), and this cortisol undermines their brain development—development in the parts of the brain that will help them self-soothe in the future.[91] Unsoothed distress (for example, when a baby is allowed to cry unsupported for longer than a few minutes) is more than your baby's current brain can handle. At this age, even a little stress can throw your baby off balance.[92]

I tell parents to wait 4 or 5 months before sleep coaching because the first several months of life are all about brain development (to make way for self-soothing) and gaining trust. Gaining trust is the building block to creating secure attachment and the development of emotional intelligence. Therefore, we focus on what we can at this stage: sleep shaping, creating supportive routines, and paying attention to feedings.

## Sleep Needs in Healthy Full-Term Babies

The typical sleep average for this second month is **10 or 11 hours at night and 5 or 6 hours during the day, spread out over several naps**—although as we learned in Month 1, there is a lot of variability in sleep needs in babies under 6 months. Current research has shown that there can be a variation of up to 8 or 9 hours in a 24-hour period for babies 6 months and under.

You may have spoken to a friend whose baby sleeps 13 hours a night, while yours sleeps only 10. Remember, that just might be the norm for your baby right now.

> Generally, newborns up to 3 months should sleep for a total of **14 to 17 hours throughout each 24-hour period**. This range includes both daytime naps and nighttime sleep. Most newborns can be awake for up to 1 hour at a time—but some for only 45 minutes.

## Night Sleep Consolidation Begins

If you have been keeping a sleep log, you may have noticed toward the end of the month that your baby has started to have one longer stretch of 4 to 5 hours of sleep at night. Yes, they will still wake frequently after this stretch—you can expect them to wake every few hours for a feeding until their typical wake-up time for the day—but celebrate this first long period of sleep!

"Sleeping through the night" is traditionally defined as a continuous stretch of sleep between 12 AM and 5 AM when there is no need for parent intervention (either soothing or feeding).[93] We start to see consolidated sleep in babies between 6 weeks and 3 months, but keep in mind that even by 9 months studies suggest that only 50 to 80 percent of babies sleep through the night on a regular basis.[94]

## Napping

At this stage, infants can stay awake for only 1 to 1½ hours before needing to sleep again. Daytime sleep is not yet organized (that is, naps are still at irregular times and are irregular lengths), but we'll give you some tips to help your baby get restorative daytime sleep even before they start napping at regular times.

## How Long Can Your Baby Be Awake?

It helps to pay attention to your baby's *window of wakefulness*, which is the length of time they can stay awake before getting overtired and fussy (and then very fussy).

If you're logging your baby's sleep, the following windows of wakefulness might look familiar to you:

Nap 1: 1 hour after waking for the day

Nap 2: 1½ hours after waking from nap 1 (if nap is longer than 45 minutes)

Nap 3: about 1½ hours after waking from nap 2 (if nap is longer than 45 minutes)

Nap 4: about 1½ hours after waking from nap 3 (if nap is longer than 45 minutes)

Evening bedtime: about 1 hour after waking from a short nap 4 (under 45 minutes) or 1½ hours after waking from a longer nap 4

As you can see, when naps are shorter, your baby's awake time will also be shorter. If your baby sleeps for 45 minutes or more, they will likely be able to stay awake for 1½ hours. If they sleep for less than 45 minutes, they may be able to stay awake for only 45 minutes to 1 hour.

Many babies are awake for a shorter amount of time in the morning, after which the time between naps remains fairly consistent for the rest of the day. The trick is to watch for tired signs while paying attention to how long your baby can naturally stay awake at this age—and then try to put them down to sleep before they become overtired (and fussy!).

## Supporting Your Baby's Sleep

### Nighttime Sleep Strategies

You're starting to see a longer stretch at night, your baby has a consistent start to their day, and you've implemented a regular bedtime routine, but are there other things you can do to support the lengthening of their nighttime sleep? Yes!

We encourage you to focus on looking for and then supporting your baby's longer stretch at night. The best way to do this is to work with where your baby is developmentally by following the Baby-Led Sleep Shaping guidelines.

#### INCORPORATE A DREAM FEED

You might experiment with *dream feeding* (also referred to as *rollover feeding*) at this stage. Your baby's circadian rhythm typically drives the deepest and longest stretch of sleep at the beginning of the night, starting at bedtime. The goal of the dream feed is to push this long stretch to their second sleep stretch of the night by regulating their first feeding, allowing you to get a good stretch of sleep, too. (Dream feeds can also be helpful during growth spurts—they can let you get extra calories into your baby without introducing an extra waking at night due to hunger.)

Here is what to do: Wake your baby between 10 PM and midnight, before you go to bed. Pick them up, nurse or bottle feed them, and then put them right back down to sleep.

Keep in mind that this works for only about 50 percent of babies. If, after 3 days, you find that doing the dream feed just adds another waking and feeding, then stop and allow your baby to take their longest stretch at the beginning of the night.

## Daytime Napping Strategies

### Is There Such a Thing as Too Much Daytime Sleep?

It is true that for some babies, getting too much daytime sleep can result in a loss of sleep at night. If your baby's naps are so long that they do not feed regularly enough to get the calories they need during the day, they are more likely to wake up hungry at night.

If your baby is napping so long during the day that it seems to be negatively affecting their nighttime sleep, and especially if they are sleeping through feedings, it may be a result of day-night confusion. Make sure that they get enough stimulation, light, activity, and fresh air during the day. Please review our tips for resolving day-night confusion on page 100.

---

### ☁ Sleep Lady Tip ☁

Understand that there is *no* predictability in your baby's naps at this age. Take each nap as it comes and don't worry. There's a lot of growing and changing ahead!

# THE ELEMENTS OF BABY-LED SLEEP SHAPING (MONTH 2)

(1) **CREATE A SLEEP-FRIENDLY ENVIRONMENT**
- Room-darkening shades.
- Soothing colors.
- White noise.

(2) **CREATE DAILY ROUTINES**
- At bedtime, use your consistent, soothing routine. Do this in your baby's nursery if you plan to eventually transition them there, even if you are currently room sharing.
- Create a shorter pre-nap version of your pre-bed routine.

(3) **PREVENT OVERSTIMULATION (FOLLOW THE 3 PM RULE)**

(4) **DON'T LET YOUR BABY SLEEP THROUGH A DAYTIME FEEDING (OVER 3 HOURS)**
Have your baby's last nap end 1 to 1½ hours before their bedtime.

(5) **SUPPORT YOUR BABY'S BUDDING CIRCADIAN RHYTHMS**
- Watch their windows of wakefulness.
- Dim lights at night.
- Expose them to sunshine in the morning.

(6) **REGULATE YOUR BABY'S WAKE-UP**
For example, wake them for the day at 7:30 AM.

(7) **REGULATE YOUR BABY'S BEDTIME**
Note the time that your baby usually goes to sleep at night and set that time as their bedtime.

(8) **FOCUS ON CREATING ONE LONGER STRETCH OF SLEEP AT NIGHT**
Try a dream feed to see if it helps (see page 143).

(9) **FILL YOUR BABY'S DAYTIME SLEEP TANK**
- Help them get naps any way you can: rocking, holding, pushing them in the stroller.
- Watch for their sleepy cues and avoid letting them get overtired.

## GET NAPS ANY WAY YOU CAN

At this stage, I suggest you help "fill your baby's sleep tank" by getting your baby naps any way you can.

Many families find that their baby naps well in an infant carrier or while lying on a flat, safe surface beside a parent or caregiver. If this is the case, then you might want to try this for one or two naps a day (or for all of them if it works for you and is safe). The bottom line is to focus on getting your newborn daytime sleep any way you can!

## AVOID OVERTIREDNESS

The most important thing to keep in mind about daytime sleep is that we don't want babies staying awake too long and getting overtired. Not only does it affect their mood, but it can impact their sleep quality and length both during the day and at night. It makes it more difficult for them to fall asleep for the next sleep period and causes fragmented sleep cycles, resulting in shorter or restless naps.

To prevent overtiredness, make sure to watch for your baby's sleep cues. See Month 1, page 103, for a list of what to look for. The only addition this month is that your baby might look away from you—perhaps stare at a wall—if they feel overtired.

Since daytime sleep is still not organized, your baby may be taking several long naps, or they may still be taking a number of shorter naps. If your baby consistently takes short naps, you will find that they may need to take more of them—often as many as four to seven—to avoid being overtired at the end of the day. If your baby is sleeping for longer periods of time, you will likely still find that they need three or four naps a day until they are closer to 6 months old.

Here is what you can focus on to improve nap quality and length:

✧ Keep your baby's environment calm to see if overstimulation has been causing shorter naps.

✧ Experiment with putting your baby in a cool, quiet, dim place for naps to see if that helps them sleep longer.

✧ Sometimes you can lengthen at least one nap in the day:

— Try extending a nap by soothing your baby back to sleep when they wake up. You can try shushing them, patting them, or even picking them up and feeding them.

— If your baby wakes consistently after 20 or 30 minutes, try setting an alarm so you can go in just before their usual wake time and encourage them to fall back to sleep before they fully wake. (This will be easier than waiting until they have woken up all the way.)

— If either of these approaches is not working after 5 to 10 minutes or your baby is crying, simply end the nap and try again next time.

✧ Some babies sleep better while in the same room with a parent. You can try keeping them close by in a bassinet outside of a bedroom or napping together on a safe surface.

✧ Some babies sleep better in motion. At nap time, you can try taking them for a long walk in a carrier or stroller.

✧ If they still take a short nap, make sure you keep their windows of wakefulness between naps short—just 1 hour—since a shorter nap means they can't stay awake long without getting overtired. This means they will need to take several naps, more than a baby who naps longer would.

---

### ☁ Sleep Lady Tip ☁

If you usually hold your baby during naps and want to put your baby down, but find they that they wake the minute you do:

Try holding them for at least 15 minutes after they first fall asleep, until they are sleeping more deeply, before putting them down.

Once you put them down, stay by their side. If they jolt awake, pat and shush them back to sleep. You can try this for as long as it feels comfortable (many families try for about 10 minutes before assuming that the nap is over).

Babies under 3 months often thrive quite nicely on short power naps; it is their parents that often have a more challenging time. If your baby has reflux, short naps can be common and may not lengthen until the reflux is under control or your baby is older—so you might as well hold off on lengthening strategies at this time.

## Co-Sleeping This Month

It's helpful to reevaluate how co-sleeping is working for you and your family each month.

If your baby is starting to show you that they require an earlier bedtime, you may want to have them start their night in a bassinet or co-sleeper, so that once they are asleep, you can safely leave the room until your own bedtime. This is one of the huge advantages of using a co-sleeper.

You may find that you want to continue to co-sleep at night but don't want to lie down and nap yourself every time your baby does. If so, you can start to put your baby in their bassinet or in a co-sleeper with the railing up for naps.

You may need to push your baby's bassinet or crib a bit farther away from the side of your bed to prevent sleep disruption. As you learned in the Development section, your baby's senses are becoming stronger, which means they are more likely to hear you when you come into bed at night or see you if they wake slightly and open their eyes.

### Transitioning from Co-Sleeping

If you find that co-sleeping at night is not working for your baby and/or family and want to slowly transition your baby to sleeping in their own crib, one great option is to use a co-sleeper attached to your bed, or a bassinet that is still near your bed, that you can eventually move farther away.

If you're ready to start the transition process, you can:

☆ Put your baby down asleep in the co-sleeper or bassinet at bedtime.
☆ Pick them up and do a dream feed (see page 143) when they first show signs of waking (hopefully after a longer stretch of sleep).
☆ Soothe them back to sleep.

✩    Return them to their co-sleeper.

✩    If they awaken a little bit when you put them down (or were not yet com-
      pletely asleep), you can put your hand on their back and pat and shush
      them to sleep.

If you decide to transition your baby to their own room when they are a little
older, they might then be developmentally ready to use my Baby-Led Sleep Coaching techniques (see Months 4 and 5 for more).

Toward the end of this month, if you feel you have an "easy" baby (one whose
cues are clear and who falls asleep quickly without much fuss), you can skip ahead to
next month's Sleep section and try practicing the Jiggle and Soothe method, a Baby-
Led Sleep Shaping technique that provides a bridge to sleep coaching. Remember,
you can always try and then decide to stop if you feel that your baby isn't ready.

## Your Sleep

Sleep is important for parents, too! Sleep deprivation makes it harder to make decisions and multitask, gives you a slower reaction time, and increases cravings for carbo-
hydrates and sugar. It's also the most commonly overlooked contributor to PMADs.

To help protect your sleep, psychologist Shoshana Bennett suggests splitting
night duty with a partner, family friend, or night nanny, if you can. She reminds us
that only one caregiver needs to be awake with the baby at a time (unless you have
had a C-section or have another medical issue). To get better quality sleep while
off-duty, Dr. Shosh suggests:

✩    Sleeping in a separate area, away from the baby and the adult on duty.

✩    Using earplugs and a white noise machine.

✩    Moving your clock away from the bed (if you tend to obsess about the time).

✩    If you are breastfeeding or pumping, emptying both breasts before bed
      (so you won't wake up engorged and in pain when you could be asleep).

As babies start to sleep for longer stretches and wake less frequently during
this month, some parents find that they have difficulty returning to sleeping for
longer stretches and even experience some insomnia. In this case, after ruling out
a PMAD, I recommend trying to get the best sleep you can by:

- ✨ Going to bed as early as you can and napping when you can.
- ✨ Making your bedroom a relaxing haven—use a diffuser with essential oil, keep the temperature cool, and make it a cell phone–free zone.
- ✨ Avoiding blue light 1 hour before bed. (It can help to wear orange-tinted glasses with a blue light filter during this time and use only orange or yellow night-lights.)
- ✨ Watching your caffeine intake. (Nursing mothers are often doing this already, as caffeine can make its way into breastmilk and keep baby awake as well.)

---

### Back to Work

Many parents head back to work this month. For back-to-work resources, including a childcare checklist and tips on breastfeeding for working mothers, please see SleepLady.com/Newborn SleepGuide.

---

 Feeling overwhelmed? One of our Gentle Sleep Coaches would love to help you create your sleep shaping plan and support you as you coach your baby through it! Visit FindaSleep Coach.com.

---

## YOUR SELF-CARE

Please do not skip over this section!

Yes, your baby is still not sleeping a lot, but you've gotten through the first month and are starting to put routines in place. That makes this a great time for putting routines in place for yourself as well.

## Moving Your Body

*The Postnatal Depletion Cure* author Dr. Oscar Serrallach suggests that birth mothers can often safely start to exercise around the middle of this month (we suggest checking with your obstetrician to be sure). He recommends starting with pelvic floor exercises and other low-impact activities like yoga, Pilates, swimming, and walking that can gently build back your core muscles.[95]

If you're having difficulty fitting "normal" exercise into your schedule (we get it!), try incorporating dance into your day, like Radha Agrawal did when she was a busy new mom. A part of her Joy Practice was to put on uplifting music, pick up her little one, and dance around the room. "I don't know where I'd be without my Joy Practice, especially during the early days of parenting," she says.

## Mindfulness, Relaxing Visualization, and Breathing

Meditation and mindfulness expert Emily Fletcher knows what it feels like to be an overwhelmed new mother! After a tough delivery (that didn't follow anything *close* to her plan) and breastfeeding challenges, she had to break her own rules about how and when to meditate to make sure she got the self-care she needed. Although she usually recommends two 20-minute meditation sessions a day, Emily suggests new parents just focus on getting in as many minutes as they can—even if that's while drinking coffee in the morning or as you slip into sleep in the afternoon. Emily gets it! She shares the following two activities that you can try to support yourself.

### A Mindfulness Exercise

While feeding your baby, try taking 5 minutes to really become mindful and present in the moment. Become aware of what your five senses are telling you: How does your body feel as you sit or recline? Can you feel air moving against your skin? What sounds do you hear around you? What do you see as you look down at your little one? Do you recognize a particular smell? Is there a taste in your mouth? Take this time to become present in the moment and feel your breath as you connect with your baby.

### Visualizing Yourself to Sleep

Often, new mothers have difficulty calming their bodies and mind for sleep (when they do have the time for it). Emily teaches something called the *body feeling technique*. She suggests lying in bed with your eyes closed and bringing your awareness to the most dominant sensation—without trying to change it or adjust it. Just bring your awareness to the spot, breathe it in, and let it say whatever it needs to say.

Perhaps your heart is beating fast. You are feeling anxious and worried about your sleeping baby—wondering if you need to check on them. Instead of judging the feeling, examine it. Perhaps you can imagine the adrenaline and cortisol coursing through your body. Instead of judging this, you might think, "Wow! My body is such a powerful pharmacy!"

Now scan your body again. What is the next most prevalent sensation?

As you scan, feel the weight of your body on the bed. Feel your muscles soften and get heavier—just breathe into the heaviness as you work with each new physical sensation.

This exercise can be very powerful. Emily finds that most people are asleep within 5 minutes of practicing it.

## Deep Breaths

In *Calm Mama, Happy Baby*, Derek O'Neill and Jennifer Waldburger recommend finding your center. One way to do this is through deep breathing using your diaphragm.[96]

### Calming Breath (Moon Breath)

Try this technique when you find yourself anxious, tense, or frustrated:

1. Hold your right nostril closed with your thumb.
2. Breathe in through your left nostril to a count of five. Make sure to inhale so that your upper chest fills with air.
3. Release your right nostril and hold your left nostril closed with your pinky.
4. Exhale through your right nostril to a count of six. Make sure to exhale so all the air leaves your abdomen.

As your baby's needs change, the cues they give you can change as well. Mindfulness can give you the presence to read these cues. And relaxing breathing exercises can help with self-regulation, which helps you read these new cues as well.

## Fantasy versus Reality

Psychologist Shoshana Bennett reminds us that listening to myths or our own fantasies about parenthood can create problems that wouldn't otherwise exist.

Expecting parents are sometimes told that all marriage or partnership issues will disappear once the baby is born. They are told that breastfeeding or co-sleeping (or both!) will solve a PMAD (or any other problem you may be experiencing) and that breastfeeding should be easy and come naturally (as Dr. Shosh points out, if this is the case, why are there so many lactation consultants?). All of these are myths that set completely unrealistic expectations and create an unmanageable amount of pressure on new parents.

### Gatekeeping

I suggest that new parents need to learn to say "yes, thank you" when they are offered help. This is because it's very easy for new parents to believe another myth: that they "should" (those darn "shoulds") be able to do everything on their own without any help.

*Maternal gatekeeping* is a behavior that can appear when the primary caregiver (often the mother), because they spend the majority of time with the baby, feels that only they can properly soothe and care for their little one. While the parent who spends the most time with the baby will have the most experience reading the baby's cues, it is important to trust that the baby will be well cared for by other trusted adults. Gatekeeping often starts with the primary caregiver's feelings but can be affirmed by partners and grandparents who fear that they will not care for the baby in the way that the primary caregiver wishes. It's important for everyone involved to work together to keep this perception from continuing.

What can you do to head off gatekeeping? Ask yourself, *Are my gates open? Or do I believe or communicate the perception that I am the only one who can properly care for my baby?* Share what you have noticed about your baby with your partner and other caregivers—their cues, what soothes them—then let them try noticing the cues or using the suggested soothing techniques, and give them permission to try out some of their own. Here are some additional tips from the website *The Bump*:[97]

- Actively plan to leave your baby with another caregiver to gain perspective.
- Learn more about parenting with your partner by reading a book or blog, or by taking a class together.
- Jump in or critique only when your baby's safety is at risk, rather than to indicate a preference or make a joke about your partner's funny way of taking care of your little one.
- Work to split the responsibility for caring for your little one 50-50, including at-home care plus daycare pickup and communication.

Dismissing the myth that only you can care for your little one will allow other caring adults to give you breaks and support . . . which you will need! Trying to do everything yourself leads to depletion and burnout, not to mention resentment. And who knows, they may find new and different ways to soothe your baby (not better, just different!)—giving you additional options for your soothing toolbox!

Other myths are about what parenthood "should" be like. Parents are told that life with a newborn should be the happiest time of their life. Or they are told that once the baby's born, parents' (especially mothers') needs shouldn't matter anymore.

It is completely normal to feel stressed and overwhelmed at this time, and to miss aspects of the life you used to have. It's okay to cry! Having a new baby can be challenging. That's why we encourage you to experiment with the techniques we've shared to help you take care of yourself, connect to your child, and enjoy the newborn phase as much as possible.

## CONGRATULATIONS!

You've learned a lot about your baby over the last 2 months, and especially about how to soothe them. Please remember that even if you don't succeed at deciphering your newborn's cues the first time, (1) you are responding to them, which is the most important part, and (2) you are getting more practice, which helps you get better at it.

# ONE-PAGE FAST TO SLEEP SUMMARY

**Month 2 Theme:** *This is the time to focus on adding soothing tools to your toolbox.*

## This Month

1. Aim for up to 20 or 30 minutes of tummy time, two to three times per day.
2. Keep a feeding and sleep log to look for when a daily pattern emerges, with one longer stretch of sleep between feedings at night. Your baby may then go longer between feedings in the morning and cluster feed toward the late afternoon or evening.
3. Remember that your baby is in the Period of PURPLE Crying (page 122), and that this increased fussiness is normal, due to natural developmental changes. It may seem like a lot to handle, but you'll see less fussiness next month!
4. Experiment with our list of soothing tools on page 132. Remember to only try one at a time.
5. Put in place the Baby-Led Sleep Shaping elements (page 145), including:
   - Support your baby's budding circadian rhythms.
   - Regulate your baby's wake-up.
   - Regulate your baby's bedtime.
   - Work on creating one longer stretch of sleep at night.
   - Fill your baby's daytime sleep tank.
6. Try a dream feed (page 143).
7. Commit to at least one self-care activity a day.

## What Not to Worry About

Nap lengths and sleep training in general. Remember, you are *not* creating bad habits! At this age, there's no wrong way to get your baby the sleep they need.

> For a printable PDF of this month's FAST to Sleep Summary plus helpful book bonuses, go to SleepLady.com/NewbornSleepGuide.

# Your Baby's Third Month

## *8 to 12 Weeks*

*This month, we address sleep changes and other developmental mile-stones you might be seeing now. We'll look at growth spurts, teething, feeding strikes, and food sensitivities; yet more calming and soothing strategies; and how to support your baby's emerging sleep "schedule."*

After my rough start with Carleigh and breastfeeding, by the end of her third month we'd gotten into a good rhythm. She definitely had her super fussy period in the evening during the second and third months. I remember regularly calling her dad to make sure he was going to come home on time, as the crying was challenging. But by that third month, I was also feeling like we were getting to know each other. She was starting to become a little person. I really paid attention to the more regular "schedule" that she started following on her own, and this helped me better recognize her tired cues. She was getting better at communicating her needs to me, and I was getting better at reading her!

It was around this time that we attended my nephew's christening. After church, we went back to my brother and sister-in-law's house. I ended up in the living room with Carleigh and a few other mothers with babies and children of various ages. Carleigh had been fed and was well rested, but she began to fuss and cry. One of the mothers asked if she could hold Carleigh as she had two children and remembered this fussy stage.

Several of the mothers told me that I should nurse Carleigh and insisted that was why she was crying. I looked at my watch and said, "No, she doesn't need to eat now." I didn't even get to finish my sentence before they attacked me for determining whether my baby needed to eat based on the clock. Finally, once there was a lull in the unsolicited advice, I shared with them that I looked at my watch to confirm that this was typically the time of day that she began to fuss and cry and that we had a routine that worked.

Luckily the mom holding Carleigh came to my defense. She shared that she remembered when her babies had gone through this phase and praised me for reading my baby and figuring out her patterns. But I was taken back by the judgment and, most of all, the questioning of my expertise—the assumption I didn't know what my baby wanted.

The mom holding Carleigh gave me such a gift when she supported me, and I would like to pass that gift on to you. Yes, you are learning with your baby (especially if this is your first) and, yes, you will make mistakes—you will try to feed your baby when they really need a new diaper or change them into a more comfortable outfit when they really need to be put to sleep. That's part of bonding with, and becoming attuned to, your baby.

Ultimately, I realized that *I* was my baby's expert. I would love for you to reach this realization as well—and not let anyone take that away from you.

## THE EMERGENCE OF A SCHEDULE

Everything will start to feel a bit more manageable this month. You may even have the sense that you're coming out of a fog. Perhaps it's a little easier to leave the house, you have routines down for feeding and pre-bed, and you are reading your baby's cues more and more easily.

Within the last month, you may have started to see the emergence of a longer stretch of sleep during the first part of the night (thank goodness!). This is because your baby is starting to produce and secrete their own melatonin, the hormone we release when our environment becomes dark. The hormone melatonin helps set our internal clock (our circadian rhythm) by making us feel drowsy. It tells us when to be asleep and when to be awake. This internal clock is supported by a consistent schedule of going to bed and waking up at approximately the same time each day.

You can support your baby's emerging circadian rhythm in the evening through dimming the lights and social cues such as a quieter environment that sets the stage for a soothing bedtime routine. When, instead, we keep a baby up past their natural bedtime and expose them to more light, they *stop* secreting melatonin and appear to get a second wind. (It's as if you tried to fall asleep after downing a double espresso.) Your little one will then be even more difficult to get to sleep for the night.

You can use this light trick in the morning, too. To help your baby's body (and yours!) stop secreting melatonin during the day, try opening the shades wide, turning on all the lights, and then popping outside for a walk.

As your baby's internal clock develops, you will start to see the glimmer of . . . dare I say . . . a schedule. For example, you may notice that your newborn starts to wake more consistently around 7 or 7:30 AM. In this example, your baby would be ready for a nap again around 9 AM. If you are having trouble seeing a schedule this month, we will help you figure out where to look and how to encourage and further it. Having a feeding and sleep rhythm helps bring predictability to your day, which often means a sense of calm for you and your baby.

A foundation of predictability makes returning to work a bit easier. You'll be able to tell your care provider roughly what to expect throughout the day—when your baby tends to nap and how often they eat. It makes it easier to make appointments with your pediatrician, too!

But it can also make it harder to go back to work, since things are now starting to feel a tad more normal. Your baby is starting to become more of a person, as well—more engaged with you and the world. The combination of this more reliable schedule and their "little personness" might make heading back to the office feel bittersweet.

# DEVELOPMENT

Your baby's brain and body continue to develop and change. Most of these changes will appear at the end of the month, but there are a few you might notice right away.

## *Vision, Taste, and Smell*

By 2 months of age, babies have developed about 90 percent of their vision and are able to focus on objects 8 to 12 inches from them—about the length of their arm. They can detect light and dark but can't see all of the colors yet.

This improved eyesight means they can start to track you. I remember the first time my daughter Carleigh tracked me across the room. I had put her down to move a basket of laundry across the room, and noticed her eyes were following me. *Wow*, I thought. *I am someone's mother, and I am clearly very important to her.* This tracking can affect your baby's sleep, as they may become more aware when you are in their sleep space.

Babies can also smell their parents (whether they are breastfeeding or not) when they are nearby; although both taste and smell develop in utero, they improve further at this age. They may wake more easily when they hear you in their space, as well. These changes in awareness and the upcoming changes in your baby's sleep cycles that will cause a "mini awakening" every 45 to 120 minutes can together mean that these "mini" wake-ups between sleep cycles turn into "full-blown" wake-ups, as your baby senses you in their sleep space. You might need to move their crib farther from your bed if you are room sharing.

At this stage, your baby may also have more difficulty falling asleep in a brightly lit room, so room-darkening shades can be very helpful. This applies to both naps and night sleep.

## *First Attempts at Self-Soothing*

At this age, babies will start to intentionally bring their hands up toward their face (which is also known as bringing their hands to their midline). Around this time, they start to put their fingers, thumb, and even entire fist in their mouth or grab something with both hands and bring it to their mouth[98] so they can suck on them to self-calm rather than remaining fussy or relying on a parent to soothe them (sometimes with a pacifier). This is the first step to self-soothing.

## Supporting Development for Better Sleep

According to *The Wonder Weeks*, at the end of this month, your baby will begin to enter the world of "smooth transitions."[99] Their actions will become more fluid as they gain control over more aspects of their bodies. At this age, many babies will be able to turn their head in a fluid motion, allowing them to turn away from over-stimulation, which helps keep them from getting overly fussy before sleep. They may also be able to roll from their tummy to their back with assistance, which means that they are on their way to rolling over on their own (some babies may already be there this month).

As a reminder, it's pretty standard for babies to be fussy and clingy before they go through a set of developmental changes. Just know that the new skills they are learning will make it worth it!

### Tummy Time

At this stage, your baby will start to roll with your assistance. Rolling on their own will be one of their first skills for self-soothing. But they'll need more muscle strength in their back, arms, and shoulders to help them out. Tummy time is the best way to help them develop these muscles.

In month 3, your baby can handle **up to 45 to 60 minutes of tummy time a day, broken into several sessions**. Use a floor mirror to encourage your baby to lift their head off the mat when on their tummy. They will love looking at themselves! Pick times when your baby is alert, aware, and social (but not right after feeding, so they are less likely to spit up).

Dr. Gabriela Zepeda, a pediatrician and Gentle Sleep Coach, suggests that we avoid frequent use of "containers," especially around 2 to 4 months of age, because they don't allow babies to practice using their muscles to move around. Any type of bucket seat or bouncy seat counts as a container. Instead, you can opt for more tummy time!

> ### ☁ **Sleep Lady Tip** ☁
>
> Sit or lie on the floor with your baby and make it a technology-free tummy time session. Your baby's development will stay on track, plus you'll get some one-on-one time to practice noticing their cues and be on your way to becoming an even better baby detective.

 FEEDING

## Feeding at This Age

On average, babies in month 2 **feed every 2½ to 3 hours during the day** and may go one longer stretch (between 4 and 6 hours) without eating at night. They will take **4 to 5 ounces per feeding**.

Gentle Sleep Coach Brandi Jordan, MSW, IBCLC, shares that breastfed babies may still be taking 8 feedings every 24 hours, while bottle-fed babies might have dropped one feeding at this point. She says that even more important than the number of feedings or the amount taken at each is making sure your baby is content between feedings and starting to have one long stretch of sleep at night.

## An Emerging Feeding Schedule

As we've discussed, because of the emergence of that circadian rhythm, you may now begin to experience at least one longer, more consolidated stretch of sleep between feedings at night. This stretch can be 4 to 6 hours at the beginning of the month and might even be 6 to 8 hours at the end of the month.

Remember, your baby is only going to take that long extended stretch once in each 24-hour period, so regular feedings every 2 to 3 hours during the day will help ensure this long stretch comes at night. That may mean waking your baby at the 3-hour mark during the day if feeding time approaches and they are still napping.

Your baby will experience a major growth spurt at the end of this month, so you may notice feeding patterns shifting around week 11. You may also see more broken sleep or wakings. This is normal and natural, so try not to worry. Feed them when they are hungry (following their cues) and allow them to increase their feeds as needed. This disruption might last for a few days (both day and night) before it evens out again.

If you find your baby needs to be fed every 3 hours during the day, your baby's feeding schedule may look similar to the one below. (Because your baby's nap schedule may still vary greatly, we've left out nap times and lengths.)

| | |
|---|---|
| **7 AM:** | Standard wake time; feeding and diaper change |
| | Nap |
| **10 AM:** | Feeding and diaper change |
| | Nap |
| **1 PM:** | Feeding and diaper change |
| | Nap |
| **4 PM:** | Feeding and diaper change |
| | Nap |
| | Possible cluster feedings (see page 127) |
| **7 PM:** | Feeding, diaper change, and possible bedtime |
| **11 PM–1 AM:** | Feeding, diaper change, and back to sleep |
| **3–4 AM:** | Feeding, diaper change, and back to sleep |

If your baby has already shifted to feeding every 4 hours and your doctor has signed off on this, you can adjust these times accordingly.

## Supporting Sleep through Feeding

### Dream Feed

If you are not yet seeing one longer stretch of sleep at night, you might want to consider adding a *dream feed* (more in Month 2, page 143).

Gentle Sleep Coach Heather Irvine, CLEC, shares, "Maria was a previous client of mine who just had her third baby. Owen was 13 weeks old when she came to me with questions about his sleep patterns. She particularly was concerned about his night wakings and wondered if they were a result of him being hungry or uncomfortable." Owen woke sporadically and there was no real pattern to his wake-ups.

Once Heather assessed his feeding and sleep logs, she determined that they could safely work toward one longer stretch of sleep at night. Owen's longest stretch at the time was only 3 hours. Heather suggested that Maria pay attention to her son's feeding cues and encouraged her to offer him a feeding at least every 3 hours during the day even if that meant waking him if he slept past a feeding time.

"We made sure he had a good feeding before bedtime," Heather says, "and then we put a night feeding plan in place." Since Maria went to bed around 9 PM, Heather suggested that for the next week, Maria do a dream feed and then log each night how long Owen slept after it. Maria found that he could sleep for a 4-hour stretch after his dream feed.

Over the next few weeks, Heather worked with Maria to create a plan in which she would push this dream feed later by 5 minutes each night over the course of 2

## Feedings at Night and Heading Back to Work

Depending on how your baby is sleeping at night, toward the end of this month they may wake once, wake twice, or, in rare cases, actually sleep through the night. Usually, your doctor will say that your baby doesn't need nighttime feedings if they sleep through the night on their own.

If you are heading back to work, however, you may decide to keep one or more night feedings in the schedule so as not to add too many changes at once. You may also decide to do so to ensure that they are getting enough nutrition and to keep your milk supply consistent if you are breastfeeding. This night feed can be a lovely time to connect with your baby after being separated during the day. It's okay to keep this feeding even if your baby doesn't need it. Please do what you need to do to make the adjustment to daycare smooth.

weeks (yes, Maria had to stay up a little later during this time). Following this plan, Maria was able to increase Owen's longest stretch to 5 hours. Eventually, Maria used this same plan to gradually lengthen that stretch to 6-plus hours.

Remember, the dream feed only works for 50 percent of babies, especially at this age. Sometimes the dream feed simply breaks up this first long stretch, rather than pushing it into the next stretch of sleep. If, after 3 days, you find that the dream feed isn't making a difference, stop and let your baby continue to take their longest stretch at the beginning of the night.

## Feeding Challenges

As you may have experienced with your little one already, feeding challenges can impact a baby's ability to sleep well. I encourage the families I work with to make addressing feeding challenges a priority; they can usually be easily overcome if dealt with promptly and not allowed to go on for too long. We want to make sure that when your baby is developmentally ready for more sleep shaping and even sleep coaching, a feeding challenge is not holding them back.

If you are not already, we suggest you log your baby's feedings (time and amount) and sleep (time and length) so you're able to quickly identify and start solving any issues that appear. You can combine this information with your baby's growth curve, tracked by your doctor, to help you know if there is an issue worth talking to your doctor about.

### Distracted Feeding

Heather shares that because babies are more aware of their surroundings at this age, they may also be more distractible during feeding time. Some babies have a fear of missing out and want to be part of the activity around them.

When babies do not eat as well during the day, it can lead to cluster feedings in the evenings and increased wakings at night to make up for lost calories. Distracted eating can also affect a breastfeeding mother's milk supply.

If your baby is particularly distracted during feeding, you can try moving to a quiet room to make sure that they are getting enough to eat during the daytime feedings. And if you find your milk supply is affected, make sure that you follow up with a pumping session when your baby hasn't fed well and see a lactation consultant if the poor feeding continues.

> Speaking of milk supply . . . Breastfeeding mothers need to nurse or pump at least once every 8 hours to keep their milk supply consistent. As your baby's night sleep stretches, keeping tabs on nursing will ensure an adequate supply. If you are worried about your milk supply, you might need to add a pumping session as your baby transitions to fewer feedings. Even going from two or three feedings at night to one could affect your milk supply. Talk to a trusted lactation consultant if you are worried.

## Bottle Refusal and Nursing Strikes

Some parents find at this age that their baby goes on a feeding strike—either refusing to nurse or refusing the bottle.

Feeding strikes disrupt sleep because a baby who is not getting enough nutrition during the day might turn to cluster feeding early in the night or even throughout the night. The baby might move to a *reverse cycle* where they are feeding more at night than during the day (see the next section).

Some parents experience feeding strikes when they first introduce a bottle to their breastfed baby. If you are seeing a feeding strike related to the new practice of bottle feeding, experiment with a bottle nipple that is more breast-like, or try soaking the nipple in Mom's milk for a few hours before offering it. You can try a fast-flow nipple to see if the flow makes it easier for them to eat or, conversely, a slow-flow nipple to make bottle feeding more like breastfeeding. If you find yourself with this challenge, we recommend seeing a trusted lactation consultant.

### Reverse Cycling

In *reverse cycling*, a baby starts associating nighttime with when most of their eating happens. Brandi Jordan shares that reverse cycling can happen when a baby is not getting enough nutrition during the day, whether because they are distracted while eating or because they are refusing to nurse or take a bottle.

If you find your little one eating more at night than during the day, first test to see if they are able to go 2½ hours or longer without feeding (this might be easier to gauge during the day). If they show you that they are hungry in less than 2½ hours, you may want to check your milk supply or formula amounts and work with your pediatrician or a lactation consultant to make sure that your baby is getting enough during the day.

Here are some tips to make sure that your baby gets the feeding they need during the day so that they're not waking more than necessary to feed at night:

1.  Feed in a place that is not stimulating: low lights, quiet, no television, no cell phone, etc.
2.  Try to ensure that your baby eats every 2 to 4 hours, even if they won't take or don't seem to need a full feeding.
3.  If nursing: Offer more frequent nursing sessions during the day.
4.  If bottle feeding: Offer your baby more ounces in each daytime bottle to see if they will take them in.
5.  Don't let your baby sleep or drift off mid-feeding.

 ATTACHMENT

Attachment, as you know by now, is built up over time. It isn't something that is there one day, gone the next, and then perhaps back the day after that. Even if you have an "off" day where you don't feel that you and your baby bonded, or you don't correctly interpret their needs the first time, the attachment that you've built so far does not just disappear. Attachment is "established through a pretty reliable and consistent pattern of response over time," shares Gentle Sleep Coach Macall Gordon, MA. "This doesn't mean that responses are perfect—just relatively consistent."

Macall also reminds us that this doesn't mean your child never experiences distress. It just means that you are there to step in as needed and keep that distress at a tolerable level. She says, "Attachment and growth result from what are called *interactive repairs*—meaning that even though there are times that you are not available or not totally present, and then you rejoin your child, there is growth that happens."

It's not the soothing itself that builds the attachment, but rather the act of interpreting your baby's signals.

However, just because your baby has called out for you does not mean you need to come to them immediately. You can let them know with your voice that you're on your way to them. This interaction lets them know that you've heard them and builds their trust in you. This trust helps solidify their sense of safety with you and with their sleep space and helps them sleep better during naps and at night.

Consistent routines are also key to building trust because they let your baby know what to expect next. For example, they learn that after their morning wake-up, you open their curtains and sing them a good morning song before you change their diaper and put them in clothes for the day. Your baby begins to trust that they will experience this series of events day after day.

You can take advantage of your baby's emerging schedule to double down on your commitment to routines throughout the day and evening. You'll have mini routines that you engage in before feedings and walks, during and after tummy time, and more. Keep repeating the routines that work and adjust any that leave your baby feeling fussy. We want routines to be your baby's friend!

If your baby is sleeping in their own room, the pre-night sleep routine is particularly important. It is a chance for you to solidify your mutual attachment before you separate for a longer period of time.

> By the beginning of this month, your baby has learned to smile intentionally. They soon discover that their smile can make *you* smile, and a sweet dialogue begins. Your baby is trying to get your attention. When they succeed, their face may light up, their shoulders may rise, and they might even make a delighted squeal.[100]

 ## SOOTHING

As you learn to read your baby's cues and respond appropriately, you are bonding and your baby is learning to trust you. And you are learning to trust yourself as your own personal baby expert! In this month, you will continue to add strategies to your soothing toolbox.

## Tips for Soothing Your Baby

As you revisit the soothing and calming strategies you've learned so far, remember to wait 5 minutes between soothing techniques, as *The CALM Baby Method* recommends. The pause allows your baby to process the new sensation that comes with each technique and gives them time to settle down.[101]

### Self-Soothing through Sucking

As you learned in the Development section, your baby will now occasionally be able to get their fisted hand into their mouth on their own. Over time, they will get even better at this, and their fists begin to unfurl. They may gradually experiment with sucking on their wrist, different fingers, or a thumb.

Your baby's motions may still be a bit spastic, and they will experiment throughout this month until the movement becomes more comfortable to them. If you are using a pacifier, you may even find they are using the pacifier less and their hand more.

> Worried about thumb sucking affecting the alignment of your baby's teeth? Don't! It's not an issue until their permanent front teeth come in. Dentists usually suggest weaning children off pacifiers or thumb sucking before they are 3 years old.[102]

If you notice your baby sucking on their fist, take note of their environment and look at your log. Ask yourself: How long have they been awake? When did they last eat? There may be nothing in particular to notice—they could be just entertaining themselves—but you may learn something about the situations in which they suck their fist. The room might be loud, or someone might have been too close to their face, or perhaps they are getting tired. This might be a new cue that will help you learn what type of soothing they need before sleep.

## Soothing Challenges

At the end of the third month, colic starts to resolve. If you're finding that the crying and fussy symptoms of colic are not dissipating, your baby may have GERD (gastroesophageal reflux disease) or allergies. Make sure you're aware of the signs of GERD and check with your pediatrician for a diagnosis. And please check out our suggestions in Month 1 (page 69) and Month 2 (page 126).

If your baby suffers from eczema—dry, itchy patches on the skin—their sleep can suffer due to discomfort. Please check out Month 1 (page 90) for some tips on how to help your little one if they are experiencing it.

 # TEMPERAMENT

Are you getting to know your baby? Have you begun noticing some characteristics of their unique temperament? As more of your baby's temperament emerges this month, you'll be able to incorporate this new understanding of your little one into the ways you soothe them to sleep.

Parents who come to me for sleep assistance at this age often ask, "What does temperament have to do with sleep?" My answer is, "Everything!"

As we've learned, temperament affects how well your baby is able to buffer input when needed, and this is directly linked to your baby's ability to go to sleep and stay asleep.

## Orchids and Dandelions

Many parents come to me during this month because they have an "alert" baby—one who is much more sensitive to external (and internal) input. I find that helping them understand their child from multiple perspectives helps them better support their little one.

In his book *The Orchid and the Dandelion: Why Sensitive Children Face Challenges and How All Can Thrive*, W. Thomas Boyce, MD, describes two types of children, each with different "processing systems": *dandelions* (non-alert babies) and *orchids* (alert babies).[103] If you have an "alert" baby, Boyce's work will give you even more insight into your little one as their senses increase in this month.

The vast majority of children are dandelions. Just like the plant, they are wired to adapt to a wide variety of environments—their internal fight-or-flight systems are not easily triggered, and they are able to flourish even under some stress or adversity.

Orchids are a much smaller group. If you've ever tried to grow an orchid, you know that they need a specific environment to thrive. They don't make it without *just* the right balance of light, humidity, and water. Children who have orchid-type wiring are genetically more reactive and sensitive to their environment and the circumstances around them.

A dandelion and an orchid who encounter the same experience will respond very differently. The dandelion may be able to buffer the stress that might come from it and recover fairly well. The orchid, on the other hand, may be much more deeply affected and have a much harder time bouncing back.

Gentle Sleep Coach Macall Gordon, MA, gives us some good news about these orchids. While they are more vulnerable to negative events or environments, they can actually benefit *more* from positive ones than dandelions do.

Orchid plants require extra labor, but they generate breathtaking blooms. You may have an incredibly fussy, nonsleeping baby who will eventually become exceedingly social and engaged and especially verbal. Eventually, they may be a toddler who comes up with every reason in the book for why they can't go to sleep at bedtime but can also name every species of dinosaur.

Macall's research (which confirms what I have also seen in my practice) shows that while a more intense, sensitive temperament is related to tons of sleep problems (pretty much all of them!), it's also associated with some impressive strengths, like empathy, perceptiveness, and engagement. As you struggle through sleep challenges with your orchid baby, remember that there is a pretty big bright side to their temperament.

Gretchen was (and still *is*) an orchid. She was very sensitive to light, noise, and people getting "in her face"—including her older sister. I had thought that the second baby "adjusts" to the stimulating environment that they come into, but I later learned that this is not true in the beginning, when they don't have any skills to fend off and reduce the overwhelm. It is also not true if your second baby has a more sensitive temperament that doesn't allow them to easily adjust to stimulating environments.

## Alert Babies and Sleep Shaping

I've worked with tens of thousands of parents of children with sleep problems, and I've come to believe that an alert, intense, sensitive temperament may be the dividing line between children who sleep easily and those who take a bit longer to learn.

Macall says, "The usual sleep training advice often just does not work for these little ones," whom she calls *live wires*. "Understanding how they tick can be key in getting them on board with sleep."

Some babies react less strongly to stimuli and events, and generally stay on a fairly even keel. We find that they are able to buffer out a lot of the external noise and stimulation in order to turn toward sleep.

Because alert babies have a much thinner barrier, sleep is more of a challenge. They are bombarded by sensory and other information and so have a lot more of it to manage. I always say that an alert baby's filter is wide open to the world, and they need our help to shut the world out in order to go to sleep.

My coaches and I have found that alert babies also tend to exhibit other traits that impact sleep and sleep shaping/coaching.

### Intensity

When it comes to feelings and reactions, everything is bigger with an alert baby. If they're happy, they're *really* happy. When they get upset, they get *incredibly* upset. These are the babies whose parents say, "If I don't get to them in a few seconds, all bets are off." Intensity is the key trait that throws sleep training off track. These powerhouses don't just fuss for 15 minutes and then fall asleep; it can be an hour or more of hysterical crying, for many nights in a row, without any change. It's no wonder that parents of alert babies abandon the typical sleep coaching methods—and it's why the slowest and gentlest approaches of the Baby-Led Sleep Shaping and Coaching process work best for them.

## Persistence

"Easygoing" and "flexible" are not in these babies' vocabulary; they do not give up easily on what they want (and can often outlast you!). This is an amazing trait for an adult to have, but in babies and children, it can wear parents out. It's important to know that any time you try to change these babies' familiar patterns, they are going to fight you. That's okay. Macall suggests that if you can stay present, supportive, and consistent, they will eventually accept the new pattern and settle in.

## Perceptiveness

These babies notice *everything*! This can be a valuable skill. Alert babies tend to grow into sensitive and intuitive young adults who, because they are so aware of those around them, more easily empathize with others. When it comes to sleep, however, you will need to be especially consistent because, as alert babies notice every small change, even the smallest changes in their routine or environment can be unsettling to them. Macall suggests that parents have routines that are clear and repetitive.

## Engagement

These babies are always "on" (that's why I call them "alert"). Macall says that it's like their brains are working on overdrive all the time, which means that it's very easy for them to get overstimulated and overtired. You may have noticed that if you are late for a nap, they move into their supersonic, booster-rocket second wind, where sleep becomes virtually impossible. If we weren't home for Gretchen's usual nap time, there would be *no* nap! Knowing your alert baby's windows of wakefulness and watching the clock will help keep you in front of that second wind.

## Irregularity and Unpredictability

Sometimes, alert babies have no reliable pattern to their feeding, sleep, or activity. They do things differently every day. One night, they may sleep well, and parents think, "Well, A, B, and C really worked!" Then, the next night, even when they follow the same steps, their baby is up every 90 minutes. If this is the case with your baby, it just means that you have to trust that what you are doing for sleep will work in the long run—even if you don't see consistent results every night. Your progress won't go in a straight line, so don't expect it to. Have a plan, stick to the plan, and your little one will eventually (mostly) get on board.

## Supporting Your Alert Baby

Alert babies prove just how much baby sleep and temperament are related. Intensity, persistence, sensory sensitivities, and the other alert baby traits can make for a perfect storm that not only makes sleep harder and more scarce, but also can really throw parents for a loop when it comes to sleep training. Other sleep books might say that sleep training takes only 3 or 4 days of "some mild protest," but after 2 hours of sweating and pleading and crying night after night with no improvement, you give up and just rock them to sleep—convinced that maybe you stink at parenting. Parents, it's not you. It's temperament.

> Review your baby's sleep tracker regularly, because it will help you understand how much sleep your alert baby really needs. Alert children often seem like they don't need as much sleep because their sleepy cues are not as obvious. I still suggest you aim for the recommended number of hours for their age. It helps to make sure that they get quality sleep during their naps and to continue to have a consistent, early bedtime.

I have always said that alert children have their filter to the world open wider than others, and we need to help them manage this large amount of input until they get old enough to begin to manage it on their own.

Caring for an alert baby can be challenging. Your alert baby may take longer to learn self-calming techniques and may be more sensitive to overwhelm and stimulation in their environment. Remember that you are their filter, and it is your job to read their cues, even though they may be harder to read. Stay curious and continue to SOAR!

We have to match what we're doing as a parent with who we are given as a baby. If we hold fast to the expectations we had before our baby was born, and their temperament doesn't match our expectations, we can feel resentful. Please don't be too hard on yourself if it's difficult for you to let go of your previous expectations, however. It can take some time and effort but it is worth it and will help you bond even better with your baby.

As Macall says, "I promise the silver linings are there. They really are. They just masquerade as a lot of unsettled crying and upset at first, before your live wire has the ability to drive their brain. It's like putting a new driver in a Ferrari. They just don't have the skill to manage that amount of horsepower. But eventually, they will. And then stand back. They are going to really take off!"

##  GETTING YOU AND YOUR BABY TO SLEEP

As you focus on bonding with and soothing your baby, their sleep will improve. Understanding their cues and responding in a way that takes into account their unique temperament will support their day and night sleep. But when it comes to sleep, it's also important to understand what your baby is capable of at this age.

### Sleep Needs in Healthy Full-Term Babies

The typical sleep averages for your baby in this third month are **10 hours at night and 5 hours during the day, spread out over three or four naps (or more if their naps are short)**.

- ✵ At night, you can expect your baby to wake two or three times between about 10 PM and 6 AM.
- ✵ Your baby can now be awake for up to 1½ to 2 hours at a time.

### Night Sleep Consolidation Continues

At this point (we hope!), your baby is taking one extended stretch at night, typically beginning at bedtime. Before now, your infant was sleeping and waking to feed in intervals driven by their feeding patterns. By this time, their circadian rhythm is helping to drive a regular nighttime stretch. This stretch, which you may have started to see at the end of last month, may average **4 to 6 hours**. Some babies may go a little longer, but it's rare.

As their circadian rhythm is evolving, you can help it along by implementing some predictability in nighttime routines and bedtime. We will give you more tips for encouraging this long stretch!

. After this one long stretch, your baby will probably wake in a **regular feeding pattern, every 2 to 4 hours, for the rest of the night**.

## *Napping*

As always, we want to make sure that your baby is getting enough sleep during the day so that they are not overtired at bedtime. Night sleep continues to develop at this age, but daytime sleep is not yet organized, so any sleep shaping that you're doing should be focused on bedtime. Naps are all about filling that daytime sleep tank.

We recommend getting your baby to sleep and getting them to stay asleep any way you can: in a dim, dark room at home, in a stroller or front carrier, being rocked to sleep and then held through their entire nap . . . whatever's necessary. As you are filling your baby's daytime sleep tank, focus on keeping their windows of wakefulness short so they don't get overtired, particularly if you find that your baby is currently taking short naps.

---

### Catnapping

Does your 9-week-old fall asleep for naps like a charm, only to wake up after 45 minutes? This is completely normal for a baby this age. Nap lengths can vary greatly in these early months. Yes, it would be great if your baby had regular 1½- to 2-hour naps. However, this is not always the norm.

---

*Supporting Your Baby's Sleep*

As the circadian rhythm starts to develop, nights begin to take shape. This is the first stage of sleep development and is an opportune time to begin nurturing healthy sleep habits.

We've already suggested some sleep shaping steps for your baby's first 2 months. You'll learn more sleep shaping suggestions this month. Since night sleep develops first, our focus at this time is on bedtime and supporting your baby's one long nighttime stretch, while also creating a strong foundation for sleep coaching in the future.

## Too Early for Sleep Coaching (or Sleep Training)

Parents are often afraid that they will create poor long-term sleep habits if they don't start sleep training their baby at 3 months (or even 6 weeks!). I tell them not to worry. Their baby is not yet ready for sleep training or sleep coaching. In fact, I've found that when parents start too early, they often end up having to start the sleep coaching process all over again several months later because the training didn't actually "take." This is because babies at this age are not developmentally ready; they don't have the "skills in their basket" to help them with the challenge of soothing themselves to sleep. But soon they will!

**Your baby is too young for any sleep training or an overly structured sleep or feeding schedule.**

For now, bonding with your baby by reading their cues and responding accordingly is still your most important focus. At this stage, calming and soothing can actually help link sleep cycles and nurture your baby's circadian rhythms—so it plays a very important role in supporting both current and future sleep.

# THE ELEMENTS OF BABY-LED SLEEP SHAPING (MONTH 3 AND BEYOND)

**(1) CREATE A SLEEP-FRIENDLY ENVIRONMENT**
- Room-darkening shades.
- Soothing colors.
- White noise.

**(2) CREATE DAILY ROUTINES**
- At bedtime, use your consistent, soothing routine. Do this in your baby's nursery if you plan to eventually transition them there, even if you are currently room sharing.
- Create a shorter pre-nap version of your pre-bed routine.

**(3) PREVENT OVERSTIMULATION (FOLLOW THE 3 PM RULE)**

**(4) DON'T LET YOUR BABY SLEEP THROUGH A DAYTIME FEEDING (OVER 3 HOURS)**
Have your baby's last nap end 1 to 1½ hours before their bedtime.

**(5) SUPPORT YOUR BABY'S BUDDING CIRCADIAN RHYTHMS**
- Watch their windows of wakefulness.
- Dim lights at night.
- Expose them to sunshine in the morning.

**(6) REGULATE YOUR BABY'S WAKE-UP**
For example, wake them for the day at 7:30 AM.

**(7) REGULATE YOUR BABY'S BEDTIME**
Note the time that your baby usually goes to sleep at night and set that time as their bedtime.

**(8) FOCUS ON CREATING ONE LONGER STRETCH OF SLEEP AT NIGHT**
Try a dream feed to see if it helps (see page 143).

**(9) FILL YOUR BABY'S DAYTIME SLEEP TANK**
- Help them get naps any way you can: rocking, holding, pushing them in the stroller.
- Watch for their sleepy cues and avoid letting them get overtired.

**(10) BEGIN TO MOVE BEDTIME EARLIER**
Each night, move your baby's bedtime earlier by 15 minutes until you are putting them down in their crib between 7 and 8 PM. Bedtime should be no more than 2 hours after their last nap.

## Moving Bedtime Earlier

Since night sleep develops first, our focus at this time is on bedtime and your baby's one long nighttime stretch. This is the first building block in shaping your infant's sleep patterns.

Last month you gently regulated your baby's wake time; now is the age to start regulating their bedtime. If your baby is waking up cranky from a late nap between 6 and 8 PM, then this is a sign to move their bedtime up to an earlier time. Then you'll want to work backward to calculate when to wake them from their last afternoon nap. If bedtime is around 7 PM, and your baby tends to have a 60- to 90-minute wakeful window, then you'll want to wake them from their last afternoon nap no later than 5:30 PM.

If your baby's sleep time has not naturally moved earlier, you can help them along. My team and I suggest **moving the beginning of their bedtime routine 15 minutes earlier each night until you are putting them in their sleep space (using the steps you usually do) around 7** PM.

> There are some babies who are happiest when they go to sleep later and who naturally wake later in the morning. If you've checked your sleep logs and this is your baby, you can support them by keeping them on this loose baby-led schedule.

### WHY IS BEDTIME SO EARLY?

While it's perfectly okay for you to stay up until 10 PM, most babies are simply not capable of staying awake past 7 or 7:30 PM without getting that (not so wonderful) second wind you're likely quite familiar with.

Watch your baby for early sleepy signs, and start the bedtime routine as soon as you see them, if not before. Once your baby gets overtired, elevated levels of cortisol make it more challenging to fall asleep and stay asleep. It also causes fragmented sleep cycles.

You may see the following with overtired babies:

☆    Difficulty falling asleep (often taking 40 to 60 minutes).

☆    Steady crying at bedtime (even when comforted) that can last up to 60 minutes.

☆    Waking within an hour of going to bed and needing help falling back asleep.

☆    Additional night wakings.

☆    Restless sleep.

☆    Early morning rising (before 6 AM).

☆    Poor naps the next day and poor sleep the following night.

If you put your child to sleep around 7 PM, they will have an easier time settling into sleep and less likelihood of night wakings and early rising. And you'll prevent them from falling into an overtired cycle.

---

## A Note from The Sleep Lady

I understand that because of your work schedule, nighttime may be the only time during the week that you get to see your baby. Unfortunately, keeping them up too late won't result in the quality time you're hoping for.

If you have no way around a late bedtime, I recommend **making a late afternoon/early evening nap a priority** so your baby can make it to a later bedtime without getting overtired. I have worked with a very small number of babies who were able to do this successfully, and only when the parents diligently committed to filling the daytime sleep tank and prioritizing the late afternoon nap. I ascribe some of this success to these babies' easy temperament—which I know you have no control over. So this may work, or it may not. I'm sorry to be the bearer of bad news!

## Gentle Pre-Sleep Coaching Techniques: The Switcheroo and Jiggle and Soothe

If your baby's sleep is going well and you would like to begin practicing something gentle that will get them ready for sleep coaching, we have a few options.

The *Switcheroo* is a very gentle technique you can try if you are heading back to work and need a solution for getting your baby down for naps. The *Jiggle and Soothe* helps your baby become more adjusted to their sleep space, although—while it still falls under the Baby-Led Sleep Shaping umbrella—it can feel like a bigger step.

### THE SWITCHEROO

Your baby probably has a familiar way of being put to sleep, which they have associated with going to sleep and need in order to do so—what I call a "sleep crutch." If, for example, your baby is nursed to sleep, that might be the only way they know to fall asleep—which can make naps at daycare or with a nanny difficult, if not impossible.

Sleep crutches are very normal at this age! But what if you could gently switch your baby to a new way of going to sleep without going so far as sleep coaching (which your baby is not yet ready for)?

The *Switcheroo* is a small preparatory technique you can try to *switch* your baby's sleep associations. It expands your baby's repertoire of ways to fall asleep, which is helpful—even critical—if you need another caregiver to put them to sleep (or if you're a nursing mother and would just like to get a break from the sleep crutch of nursing your baby to sleep).

Let's say your baby is currently used to being nursed to sleep. To perform the Switcheroo, you would nurse them almost asleep, then pass them off to another caregiver, who could then rock them to sleep completely before putting them down in their sleep space. Yes, you are creating a *new* sleep crutch—being rocked to sleep—but this one doesn't require a nursing mother.

A similar switch is from nursing to bottle feeding. You can follow your standard pre-sleep routine and then offer your baby a bottle to feed to sleep that way. Now you have a baby who can be fed to sleep by other caregivers.

# BABY-LED SLEEP SHAPING AND COACHING™

A gentle approach led by your baby's unique temperament and needs.

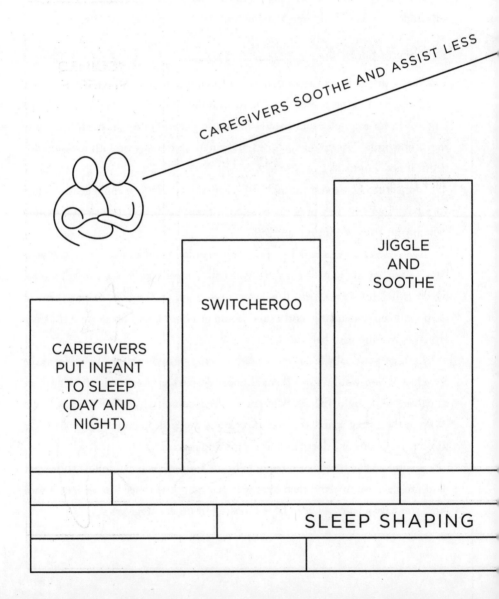

CAREGIVERS SOOTHE AND ASSIST LESS

JIGGLE AND SOOTHE

SWITCHEROO

CAREGIVERS PUT INFANT TO SLEEP (DAY AND NIGHT)

SLEEP SHAPING

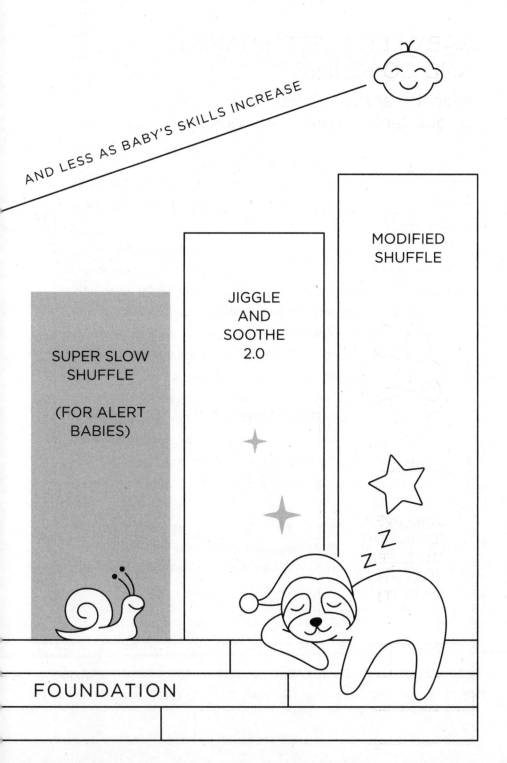

AND LESS AS BABY'S SKILLS INCREASE

MODIFIED
SHUFFLE

JIGGLE
AND
SOOTHE
2.0

SUPER SLOW
SHUFFLE

(FOR ALERT
BABIES)

FOUNDATION

An added benefit of the Switcheroo is that your baby will be less attached to the association you swap in because it is so new. In the future, when you and your baby are both ready for sleep coaching, this new association may then be easier to drop than their original association.

---

## The Alert Baby Switcheroo

What if you have a particularly alert baby, but would still like to try the Switcheroo? You can modify the steps to be even more incremental.

Eleven-week-old Jasper was able to fall asleep for naps only if he was rocked in a baby carrier for what felt like for hours at a time. For his parents, I designed a very gradual approach. First, his father completed the standard step of rocking Jasper to sleep by walking him in the baby carrier. Second, I had his father slowly and gently unhook each side of the carrier while supporting Jasper with his hands. Third, his father *very slowly* lay down on the bed with Jasper's legs still in the carrier. Over the course of a few more minutes, the carrier was unhooked from around the father's back but still kept on Jasper as he lay on the bed, with his father lying down with him. Once he was in a deep sleep, the parents *very* slowly and gently transferred him into his crib.

Eventually, they were able to complete this process in half the time. And soon after that, they were able to move to the Switcheroo itself: rocking him to sleep for naps and then placing him in his crib, to which Jasper responded quite well.

---

THE JIGGLE AND SOOTHE

If it feels like things are starting to fall into place in the sleep department and your baby may be ready for the next step, I suggest something I call the *Jiggle and Soothe*.

☁ **Sleep Lady Tip** ☁

Don't worry if you are using strategies such as nursing, rocking, or comforting your baby to sleep if it is what is working for you right now.

These aren't necessarily bad habits, and they can easily be phased out when your baby is older and more capable of learning how to sleep more independently.

The Jiggle and Soothe is not a sleep coaching method, but it will help to prepare your baby (and you) for gentle sleep coaching in the next couple of months. At this age, I recommend you practice this step first at bedtime.

To practice the Jiggle and Soothe:

1. Put your baby down in their sleep space already asleep. This means that you can use whatever soothing methods you've been using (feeding, rocking, shushing, patting, etc.) to help your baby get there.
2. Once you lay your baby down in their bed, gently jiggle their chest a little bit. (I call this "jiggling the burrito," because if your baby is still swaddled, they look like they are snugly folded into a tortilla like a baby burrito.) The jiggling will cause your baby to wake a little, open their eyes, and hopefully recognize where they are (in their sleep space).
3. Pat and shush your baby to get them back to sleep.
4. If your baby wakes fully or becomes upset, pick them up and comfort them back to sleep.
5. Try again the next night, to get them used to the process.

If your baby is responding particularly well to the Jiggle and Soothe, you're welcome to page ahead to Month 4 and try some of the more advanced Baby-Led Sleep Shaping tips we share there. But again—don't worry if they are not yet ready!

## Why We Start at Bedtime

Bedtime is the easiest time to sleep shape and sleep coach because as darkness comes on in the evening, it cues your baby's body to produce the hormone melatonin. Melatonin makes their body feel drowsy. This, plus the sleep pressure that has been building in them throughout the day, makes it easier for your baby to fall asleep.

Some families focus on sleep coaching at bedtime only for a long time. At wakings the rest of the night, and also during naps, they do whatever they need to (feeding, rocking, holding) to get their baby to sleep. Once their baby is able to put themselves to sleep at bedtime, they move on to using the method during other nighttime wakings and then eventually for naps.

What we want is for your baby to make that little bit of progress that lets you say, "Oh! It's working!" so that you feel empowered and have faith in the process—and your baby's skills. Then we can add additional steps, like addressing night wakings (which we'll discuss in Months 4 and 5).

## Modifying the Baby-Led Sleep Techniques

Please don't despair if your baby isn't ready for the version of each method I describe, in this month or future months. You can break any technique we've suggested into multiple baby steps to make them very gradual and even more gentle. You can (and I'd argue *should*) modify the methods to work for you and your baby. Modifications are part of the foundation of Baby-Led Sleep Shaping and Coaching, as you want the process to be led by your baby's unique temperament and needs. And especially if your baby is a bit more alert than most, modifications will be the name of the game.

## Co-Sleeping This Month

If you are bedsharing, a few things may change this month that have implications for your baby's naps:

- ✄ **You may not wish to nap when your baby naps,** so you might want to transition your little one to a crib or a bassinet for naps.
- ✄ **A nanny or other caregiver may start watching your baby during naps**, so you may want to get your baby used to napping in a spot other than your bedroom.
- ✄ **Your baby may start rolling** (a skill gained around 12 weeks), which means a sleep surface without four open sides is no longer a safe option.

You needn't worry about creating bad habits at this stage, but you'll also want to consider how what you are doing now is different from what you'll do in the future. If you don't plan to co-sleep with your baby for much longer, you'll want them to become comfortable in the long-term location you've chosen for them. You might start the transition process to a crib by having your baby nap in it during the day so that it's not a completely foreign space whenever you choose to move them there permanently.

If you're looking for guidance on weaning your little one from co-sleeping, please see our suggestions in Month 4.

## Sleep Challenges at This Age

You've read the sleep expectations for this age and know that your baby is unlikely to sleep through the night this month. If you are struggling through sleepless nights with your little one, our main suggestions are to double down on our sleep shaping guidelines and try out either the Switcheroo or the Jiggle and Soothe. But there are a few other sleep challenges you may also be facing this month.

### Not Seeing the Long Stretch at Bedtime

If you're not yet seeing that one longer stretch at night, please go back over the sleep shaping guidelines on page 178 to make sure that you've implemented each of them. These elements are specifically recommended to help your baby develop this longer stretch.

Another solution is to try a dream feed, which is also designed to promote that long stretch. Please see the dream feed tip on page 143.

 ## Swaddle Weaning

If your baby is not yet rolling, you can continue to swaddle them. If they are rolling, however, you'll want to wean them from the swaddle. You can go "cold turkey" and just stop using the swaddle outright or you can try a more gradual approach.

To gradually wean your baby from the swaddle, begin by wrapping them as you have been, but leaving one arm out. If this goes well with one arm, you can move to having both arms out and merely wrapping the swaddle around your baby's chest to provide comfort. This transition can also be made using a sleep sack with removable arms, following the same process; there are lots of sleep sacks that are tight about the trunk of the body, too.

Even if you choose the cold turkey approach to swaddle weaning, I recommend using a sleep sack with removable arms. You'd simply use the sack without the arms right away, rather than going through a transition process where you remove one arm at a time.

Please see my website for suggested swaddling products: SleepLady.com /Products.

Whenever you make a change in your baby's sleep routine, be prepared for them to be frustrated, upset, and cry. Make sure you're making this change after a day of good naps and their standard pre-sleep routine. If you have a sensitive baby that really likes the comfort of the swaddle, you might want to use the Switcheroo

 Feeling overwhelmed? One of our Gentle Sleep Coaches would love to help you create your sleep shaping plan and support you as you coach your baby through it! Visit FindaSleep Coach.com.

by holding them to sleep in the sleep sack. Just be prepared for them to wake more frequently during this transition.

## YOUR SELF-CARE

Have you been able to commit to several hours of "off-duty" time each week, as we suggested in the first chapter? It may seem like you have no time for self-care lately, but that is exactly when it is most necessary.

In his work on postnatal depletion, Dr. Oscar Serrallach suggests that we also look at our drive for perfectionism. This drive can push us into the unhealthy role of the "martyr" in relationship to our baby and family needs.[104] I see this in my clients all the time. They want to give their babies what they need, but feel that they have to do everything themselves because it has to be done perfectly. This mindset is very normal! But unfortunately, it just leads to even more stress. Try to look at the situation differently and remind yourself that taking care of yourself *is* taking care of your baby. Supporting our physical and mental health is wonderful for our families.

---

### PMADs

Please make sure that you and your partner are keeping your eyes out for signs of postpartum mood and anxiety disorders. If you see even the slightest sign, check with a trained professional. (If you need help finding one, see PSIDirectory.com.) There is no reason to suffer when there is help out there!

---

### Walking Mindfulness

Because things can be so busy with a newborn, I encourage you to give yourself self-care *while you are with* your baby. Meditation expert Emily Fletcher suggests a mindfulness exercise that takes no extra time out of your already busy day, because it's combined with something you're already doing: getting your baby out of the house for a walk! Mindfulness is a great way to help you feel calm and grounded . . . even if it's just for a few minutes.

As you take your baby for a walk, become particularly mindful of each step. Can you feel your right foot as it touches the ground? Your left foot? Start breathing in conjunction with your footfalls.

Slowly count as you breathe: *in, two, three, four*, then *out, two, three, four.*

Continue to practice hyperpresence. You might think, *Look, my hands are on the stroller. Now I am looking at my baby. My left foot is hitting the ground.* Step by step, you are practicing muscle presence. Ask yourself: What you are noticing?

This practice will help you destress. It will also allow you to feel more present, which contributes to your ability to bond with your baby and effectively read their soothing cues. When we are more present, we are also calmer. And a calmer parent makes for a calmer baby!

## Your Self-Care Schedule

Consider integrating your own daily self-care routines with the routines you've created for your baby. Here are some self-care practices you can add to your schedule:

- ✡ If you can, get your baby and yourself 15 minutes of sun exposure between 8 and 10 AM. This will not only set both your internal clocks, but also trigger the production of vitamin D, which helps regulate mood and reduce depression.[105]

- ✡ Turn on a song and dance around the room with your baby. Or dance with your baby in a carrier while doing a task—like unloading the dishwasher or doing laundry.

- ✡ Take a restorative yoga class online or in person—with Mama and Baby yoga, you can bring your baby along.

- ✡ See an acupuncturist (some can perform acupressure on your baby, too!).

- ✡ Do pelvic floor exercises while your baby is doing tummy time.

- ✡ Connect with your partner and talk about the type of parents you want to be as you snuggle your baby together.

In this day and age, it is a cliché to hear that parents need their own self-care. But we hope that you are starting to understand how integral your health is to not only your baby's health, but their sleep as well. Lack of sleep can make this a very stressful time for you. This stress is picked up by your baby, and it can make them more difficult to soothe and put down to sleep. Finding places where you can add regular self-care will support your sleep and, in turn, your baby's.

## NEXT MONTH

There are positive changes coming ahead—but first, there's the 4-month sleep regression. While it may feel challenging to support your baby through this phase, the result will be even better sleep in the future. I'll help you navigate this stage in the next chapter.

## ONE-PAGE FAST TO SLEEP SUMMARY

**Month 3 Theme:** *More calming and soothing strategies will help support your baby's emerging sleep "schedule."*

### What to Focus on This Month

1. Aim for 45 to 60 minutes total of tummy time per day spread across a few sessions. This is a great age for a play mat with colorful toys that they can reach for.

2. Remember that your baby is going to take only one extended stretch without eating in each 24-hour period, so feeding them every 2 to 3 hours during the day will help ensure this long stretch comes at night. That may mean waking your baby at the 3-hour mark during the day if feeding time approaches and they are still asleep.

3. Make your back-to-work transition plan, if you are going back to work this month (see the appendix).

4. Put in place the Baby-Led Sleep Shaping elements (page 178), including:
   • Begin to move bedtime earlier.

5. Pay attention to whether your baby is rolling over.

6. Read about the Switcheroo (page 181) and Jiggle and Soothe (page 184) to see if you want to try out either of these Baby-Led Sleep Shaping approaches.

7. Create a self-care schedule.

### What Not to Worry About

Night weaning, sleep coaching, or nap coaching. Your baby is not ready yet!

For a printable PDF of this month's FAST to Sleep Summary plus helpful book bonuses, go to SleepLady.com/NewbornSleepGuide.

# Your Baby's Fourth Month

## *12 to 16 Weeks*

*This month, you'll learn about the 4-month sleep regression and what you can do to soothe your baby through this time. You'll also be introduced to the Baby-Led Sleep Coaching Readiness Checklist to see if your baby is ready for some gentle sleep coaching steps. If they are, we'll offer a few things you can try.*

### Parent Spotlight: Ann
*Parent of a 14-week-old daughter, Sydney*

I used to feed Sydney to sleep and then back to sleep again when she woke, which often was twice a night. She used to take "decent" naps, and I thought I was truly blessed with an angel baby.

Then, just before she turned 4 months old, everything fell apart! She wouldn't fall asleep eating, or if she did, she woke the second I put her down and then proceeded to wake several more times during the night. She seemed fussy all the time and constantly wanted to feed. I was so nervous because I had planned to return to work soon, and I wouldn't be able to function like this. I also couldn't imagine how daycare would deal with her.

From Kim, I learned that Sydney was likely going through the 4-month sleep regression—a big developmental milestone. This explained a lot! Kim helped me focus on what I could control: being consistent with my soothing routines, responding to Sydney's feeding and sleep cues, and increasing feedings during the day to make sure that it wasn't hunger keeping her up at night. I soothed her and helped her to sleep until she was through the regression, which took a week or so. I worked hard to keep her from getting overtired or hungry and responded to her needs quickly.

Once we were on the other side, Kim laid out a plan to improve Sydney's sleep with some timing tips, an early bedtime, and a night feeding plan (so we got back down to only two feedings a night instead of four to six!). Once I was ready, we started putting Sydney down at bedtime with Jiggle and Soothe 2.0. [Sleep Lady note: We'll teach you this later in this chapter!] At first, she cried more than I was comfortable with, so we stopped and waited a week. When we tried again, I put her down, stayed by her side, and soothed her to sleep. I was doing a lot of shushing and patting, but at least I wasn't spending an hour feeding and holding her to sleep only to have her wake the second I put her down. I slowly reduced my patting and just shushed.

After a few days, I reduced that, too, until I could see that she was really putting herself to sleep on her own. She would rub the back of her head against the mattress, roll to her side, and conk out. A miracle! I focused on bedtime at first, waiting until she got a little older before we addressed naps or nighttime feeding. I felt so empowered! Kim laid out a gentle plan that resonated with us and gave us hope. We could do this!

## WHAT HAPPENED TO MY BABY?

Oh, dear! Here we had you excited about schedules and long sleep stretches, and now some (or a lot!) of that might have gone out the window. For most families, the 4-month sleep regression feels like their baby is taking a step back when it comes to sleep, losing all the progress they had been making.

We get it!

My Gentle Sleep Team is here to help you to understand what your baby is going through, and help you create the foundation for better sleep in the future. With a little extra planning and tailored tools, your baby's response to this development stage doesn't have to turn your life (and sleep) completely upside down any longer than it takes your baby to get through this milestone.

## DEVELOPMENT

Your baby is experiencing intense physical and neurological growth this month. Those consistent routines you worked so hard on last month and the month before may not work like they used to, and your baby's sleep is likely to be disrupted. And this particular developmental phase can last longer than the previous ones—from 1 all the way up to 6 weeks![106]

Changes in brain and body development tend to cause behavioral changes (including sleep changes), and this can—understandably—be very frustrating to parents! When parents aren't aware of what's going on with their baby developmentally, they can also get pretty worried.

Your baby is beginning to develop depth perception and will go through a burst of new cognitive awareness—they are starting to understand what is going on around them. Building on last month's development, this month brings increased senses of smell, sight, taste, hearing, and touch into their world.

At this point, your baby will start to make more intentional movements and sounds. They are able to see a toy that they want, reach for it, and grab it. They can then turn it around, pass it to their other hand, or put it in their mouth.[107] This is an especially helpful development if your baby is soothed by a pacifier. Although it won't happen this month, they will eventually be able to reach for a fallen pacifier and bring it back to their mouth on their own. Yay! On the safety side, however, you'll now have to keep a closer eye on their surroundings because they might grab something sharp or a hot cup of coffee without understanding the danger.

Your baby might make more attempts to roll at this age.[108] Maybe they have already succeeded and are trying to replicate the move, or maybe they are trying to do so for the very first time. Remember that rolling will be part of your baby's sleep self-soothing toolbox. When they want to change positions, they'll be able to do so themselves rather than needing your help.

At this stage, babies have learned to push a bottle or breast away from their mouth when they are full.[109] They can now use movement alongside their other cues to give you a better idea of what they are trying to communicate. You still need to keep your magnifying glass out, though! When your baby pushes a bottle or breast away, it could mean that they are full . . . or it could be that they are simply distracted. Your baby is more aware of their surroundings than ever and more easily distracted by them. I often remind parents that pushing a breast away doesn't mean that they need to start weaning their baby.

Your baby will also start to recognize their own name around this time. Once they do, your communication with them really kicks into high gear!

According to *The Wonder Weeks*, your baby is now going through a major developmental leap, and as with other leaps, this explains their fussiness, moodiness, and clinginess. You may find them wanting more of your attention and cueing you for more touch, holding, and entertainment.

These new skills let your baby start learning cause and effect, as well as object permanence (more on this next month). They may use their voice to squeal, laugh, cough, or cry just to elicit certain responses from you. A hint of shyness or anxiety about strangers may also begin to set in at this stage, and your baby may want to stay close to you and your partner. Even other family members such as grandparents may elicit a meltdown when your baby leaves the comfort and safety of their parents' arms.

## The 4-Month Sleep Regression

**Sometime between weeks 14 and 17, your baby may go through what is commonly called the 4-month sleep regression**, a period of unusually excessive fussiness and sleep disruption. Please keep in mind that not all babies experience a sleep disruption. But my main focus for the month will be helping parents whose babies do experience disruption navigate the regression.

The 4-month sleep regression has two "causes." The first is the physical and neurological developmental changes you learned about above. Any time a baby experiences physical and neurological development, sleep is often disrupted. These types of developmental changes regularly cause extra fussiness and clinginess and can make it harder for your baby to go to sleep in the first place.

The second cause of sleep disruption this month is a change in your baby's sleep cycles. When your baby was first born, they spent equal time in REM sleep and non-REM sleep. This month your baby is beginning to enter the adult world of sleep, which means that they will start cycling through four very distinct sleep stages, just like you: two light stages of sleep, deep sleep, and REM sleep.[110]

In the past, your baby might have been a bit restless at the beginning of each sleep stretch, but once they transitioned to their non-REM sleep stage they slept soundly. Now, instead of going from just one sleep stage (REM sleep) to a second (deep sleep), they are cycling through four. This cycle is new to them, but to make matters worse, they are now also partially waking whenever one sleep stage ends, before the next begins (which is an additional sleep change that occurs this month). Imagine not knowing how to put yourself to sleep, and then finding that you are suddenly waking and needing to fall back asleep multiple extra times a night.

In other words, not only is your baby experiencing a developmental change (which will often negatively affect sleep regardless of the type of change involved), but this developmental change is directly related to how they experience sleep. This is the 4-month sleep regression in a nutshell.

## Supporting Willow's Sleep Regression

When 14-week-old Willow was in the throes of the 4-month sleep regression, she seemed cranky and fussy more often than not. She fought sleep and pushed away her bottles. Her parents weren't using consistent routines to help prepare her for sleep, which made both the transition and sticking to a regular bedtime difficult. However, when they *could* get her to sleep for naps (even if it had to be in her stroller), she napped well. The same went for her nighttime sleep. Once she finally got to sleep, she woke only once for a feeding (which was great!). But her nap times and bedtimes were all over the place, which meant that she was getting an inconsistent amount of sleep each day.

I recommended that her parents track her sleep and feedings. We then regulated her bedtime to around 7 PM each evening. And I suggested that they start to gently regulate her nap times as well.

Willow's first nap often came around 90 minutes after her morning wake-up, and if they let her sleep as long as she wanted, she could happily sleep up to 3 hours. This long nap would then wreak havoc on her afternoon naps—either she wouldn't go to sleep easily, or she'd nap so late that it would throw off her usual bedtime. This resulted in days where she would have only two naps and be exhausted by bedtime. Her parents thought that by following Willow's lead, all would fall into place; however, the opposite ended up happening.

We reviewed her sleep log together and made a plan to put her down for her daily naps at more consistent times: around 9 AM, 12 PM, and 3 PM each day. Her parents had her nap in her stroller, as that worked best for their family. I told them to be prepared for this to stop working; in my experience, a sleep crutch like this may work for a little bit, while parents are working on night sleep shaping and coaching, but ultimately, how long its effectiveness lasts is based on the baby's temperament. At that point, they'd need to do some nap coaching—which would likely be easier if Willow was already starting to put herself to sleep independently at bedtime. The nap coaching would just need to address Willow learning to go to sleep without the movement of the stroller. But at this stage, we were focused on filling the daytime sleep tank however we could!

Willow's parents had been giving her a bottle right before her pretty late bedtime. Because she was overtired by this point, rather than accepting it, she would refuse to eat. When her parents took a little extra time to recognize her cues, they realized that she had been saying, "I'm sleepy. Just put me down."

They had also been trying to feed her both before her naps and immediately when she woke up from them. In other words, they were feeding her as frequently as they had when she was younger—but at this age, she wasn't yet hungry, because her bigger tummy allowed her to eat more at each feeding. Her parents had been missing both her sleepy cues and her hunger cues. Once we reviewed the sleep and feeding tracker together, they were able to see this pattern for themselves.

Here is a breakdown of what was happening: During the peak of the regression, Willow was having a harder time getting to sleep, leading her parents to struggle to put her down. When she cried, her parents would do more and more to try to soothe her, and she would get overwhelmed. They finally figured out that to get her to go to sleep successfully, they needed to do less: put her down at a consistent time after a soothing routine and just stay by her side to calm her. As a result, Willow started figuring sleep out for herself.

Willow had been born slightly early and with torticollis (which meant her neck was tilted to one side and she experienced muscle spasms), for which she received physical therapy. As a result, she was slow to roll (and later crawl), but once she did start to roll—initially just to her side—she was less cranky and able to put herself to sleep more independently at bedtime. She then slept until her one feeding and went back to sleep until morning.

In the end, the family got themselves on a gentle schedule where Willow napped well in her stroller three times a day—her daytime sleep tank was kept full! They also increased tummy time to help her learn to roll over completely, knowing this might take longer given her still-under-treatment torticollis, and were excited when she reached that milestone, because it meant she'd soon be able to soothe herself at night by getting into a more comfortable position. There was light at the end of the tunnel!

## Supporting Development for Better Sleep

Ultimately, the physical and neurological developments that occur this month are what will get your baby to the point where they are able to soothe themselves and fall asleep on their own. It's just a rocky road to get there! In the meantime, the best way to support them is to help with their physical development—and that means tummy time.

## Tummy Time

In month 4, your baby can handle **up to 90 minutes of tummy time a day, broken into several sessions**. As always, pick a time when your baby is alert, aware, and social (but not right after feeding, so they are less likely to spit up).

Sometimes both parents and babies are sick of tummy time by this month. I remind them that the whole point of tummy time is to put our babies in a position they don't normally find themselves, so that they will build muscles and learn skills that will help them later learn to roll, crawl, and eventually walk.

Your baby might feel uncomfortable and get frustrated during tummy time. Some babies *really* let you know that they don't like tummy time! It's tempting to give them a pass and skip it for the day. But while your baby might not like what is happening at the moment, it will help them in the long run.

This is a good opportunity to reframe the tummy time experience as one of many dances you will do with your baby to let them feel a little frustration. (You will go through something similar as you engage in the Baby-Led Sleep Coaching steps.) When they fuss, rather than immediately ending the session, you can put a light hand on their back and verbally console them so that they know you are there and supporting them. You can say, "Yes, I'm sure this feels frustrating. You're not used to being in this position, are you? But you're not alone. I'm here with you." As you reassure them, you can count to 20 to lengthen tummy time just a little while also reassuring your baby through this frustrating moment.

One of the first signs that tummy time is "working" is when your baby rolls over on their own. That is what you both are working toward!

The parents of 15-week-old Elizabeth told me, "We felt like we had a new baby once she could roll." Elizabeth was an alert baby who, once she mastered rolling both ways, would sleep in the corner of her crib, covering her face with her arms, or with her face smooshed up against the mattress to block out the outside world. "At first, she would roll over on her tummy. It would stress us out, but we reminded ourselves that we had a safe sleep space with no bumpers and a breathable mattress."

The commitment to tummy time really paid off. "The first time she rolled, Elizabeth seemed pretty shocked! Her shock quickly moved to a sense of empowerment once she tried a few more times." Elizabeth's parents realized that their daily tummy time sessions had helped her learn to handle small (and eventually larger) bits of frustration.

> If you're not seeing progress toward rolling, did you know that you can actually teach your baby how to roll at this age? For tips and a video on how to do this, please see Pathways.org /When-Can-Baby-Roll-Over-Tips-To-Help-Baby-Roll/.

 ## FEEDING

Feeding habits may seem to regress this month, along with sleep. Babies may be more distracted while feeding in the daytime due to their increased awareness of their surroundings. They may have shorter, more frequent feeds and need additional feeds in the night when going through this stage. While this is often due to them feeding less during the day, they may also just need more calories for growth and development. With all the changes in feeding and sleep, it may feel like you have gone back to the newborn stage!

### Feeding at This Age

On average, babies **feed every 2½ to 3 hours (some up to 4 hours) during the day** and may go one long stretch (4 to 6 hours) without eating at night. By the end of this month, some babies can sleep for an 8-hour stretch without feeding. They will take **4 to 6 ounces per feeding**.

Feeding amounts will depend on how long your baby sleeps at night and how frequently they eat during the day. If their feedings reduce during the night, they may need to feed more during the day.

A shift in appetite as a result of the 4-month developmental milestones may cause nursing mothers to experience a drop in milk supply. If you experience this, you can add an evening dream feed before you go to bed to make sure your baby is getting enough calories (and also try to get that nice long stretch of sleep together with your baby).

## The Myth of Solid Food and Sleep

Parents regularly ask me if offering their baby solid food now will help them sleep better at night. The answer is that research doesn't support the idea that solids promote better nighttime sleep. A study in the *New England Journal of Medicine* found that feeding rice cereal early to babies did not help them sleep longer. In fact, it found that babies who were fed rice cereal before 4 months of age slept *less*.

The reason the myth that feeding your baby solids will help them sleep longer at night persists is that sometimes it does work—just not for the reasons that you think. If the baby is distracted and not eating well during the day, they don't feel full at night and this can impact sleep. Sometimes, if they are given a bottle with rice at night, they might sleep longer. But the real issue is that they are not getting enough milk or formula during the day.

Cereal is also linked to obesity in babies—another reason to manage the real issue of low feeding during the day, rather than try to treat the symptoms with solids.

My team discourages parents from starting solids simply for sleep reasons. At this age, breastmilk and formula are still your baby's best source of nutrition. To determine the best time to start on solids, work with your pediatrician.

## Supporting Sleep through Feeding

As you support your baby through the 4-month sleep regression, think of feeding as something you can adjust to encourage the sleep that they *are* getting.

### Supporting Nighttime Feedings

At this age, it is completely normal for your baby to be waking during the night for one to three feedings between bedtime and morning wake-up. Don't be discouraged if you find that your baby, who had previously been able to sleep for a 6- to 8-hour stretch, is all of a sudden waking more to feed. They are growing rapidly and going through a lot of development, so they really do need to eat. (That said, we want to help you get back that long stretch in the night, and we want to keep your baby from slipping into reverse cycling—see below.)

Soon enough, you will miss those quiet night feedings. No, really!

As long as your baby is still eating during the night, it's important to maintain a sleep-friendly environment. During night feedings, make sure that you keep the room quiet and dark and cause as little disruption as possible. Doing this will gently remind your baby that nighttime is for sleep, not play.

You'll know if your baby needs to feed at night by sharing your feeding log with your pediatrician and lactation consultant. If your baby is not hungry in the morning, then you can work on reducing their nighttime feedings. Even snacking when they wake in the middle of the night, instead of taking a full feed, is a sign that night feedings may no longer be necessary—or can at least be reduced.

This might also be a sign that your baby is ready for some gentle sleep coaching at night (check out the Baby-Led Sleep Coaching Readiness Checklist in the Sleep section of this chapter and read more about how and when to start).

## Not Seeing the Long Stretch of Sleep? Try a Dream Feed

If you are not yet seeing this long stretch we've told you about, a dream feed might help. A dream feed can help to reset the clock, stretching out the time before their next feed and making that their *long* stretch of the night. For more on dream feeds, see Month 2 (page 143).

Did you see this long stretch last month but now, with the 4-month sleep regression, it has disappeared? If so, please hold tight until you feel that the sleep regression has passed. Then check out the Sleep section of this month for how to bring this long stretch back.

## Feeding Challenges

If you and your pediatrician haven't diagnosed or addressed a lingering feeding challenge, this is the time to do so. You'll want to make sure that your baby's feeding is on track before practicing the Baby-Led Sleep Coaching I recommend at the end of this chapter and in the next.

### Reverse Cycling

You learned about *reverse cycling* last month. If you suspect that your little one is starting to reverse cycle, please return to this section in Month 3 (page 166) to get tips on how to prevent it from continuing.

A dream feed can also help with reverse cycling, as it will help you get your baby the extra calories they may have missed during the day.

 ## ATTACHMENT

Your main focus this month is soothing your baby through the 4-month sleep regression. While you're doing this, you can continue to build attachment through daily and nightly routines and lots of snuggles and reassurance. The strong attachment and trust you've built over the last 3 months, and continue to reinforce this month, will help Baby-Led Sleep Shaping and Coaching go a bit more smoothly in the near future.

 ## SOOTHING

When it comes to soothing, we recommend doing whatever you've found that works to get you through the 4-month sleep regression. Use the tools we've shared with you over the last 4 months, keep an eye out for the new cues you're learning during this time, and soothe your baby accordingly.

Your baby is starting to communicate their emotions through facial expressions, which means that their cues are getting easier and easier to read. You've also learned more about your baby's temperament, which you can fold into your soothing practices.

Your baby is becoming more sensitive, so soothing them effectively may actually require less intervention at this stage, instead of more. As your baby experiences the fussiness that comes with their neurological and physical development this month, experiment with different levels of soothing to see what works best (they may not respond the same way they did last month).

## Soothing and Sleep

Because your baby's senses are more heightened now, you may need to make some changes to create a more soothing, sleep-friendly environment. You may have to use room-darkening shades and set the room at a lower temperature. If you are room sharing, you may need to move their crib farther away from your bedside, since they are now more aware of your presence.

Your soothing pre-bed routine will continue to be important. You can use some of the soothing techniques we've recommended over the previous months: a warm bath (not necessary every night), massage, reading a book, rocking, patting, cuddling, and white noise. By this time, your baby can actually recognize repetition in their daily routine, so following your chosen routine, culminating with a predictable bedtime, can help them associate the routine with sleep. You can use a condensed version of this routine pre-nap.

This is a time to pay particular attention to your baby's sleepy cues so that you can respond to them as quickly as possible. Your baby still needs a nap every 1 to 2 hours (shorter naps will mean shorter wakeful windows), even if they are fighting it. Remember, if your baby is overtired, they will be more difficult to soothe and get to sleep.

 ## Pacifiers This Month

By this age, you will probably have determined whether your baby seems soothed by a pacifier. In some cases, your baby may have made the decision that they are not interested in using one, even if you are okay with it.

At this stage, we recommend using pacifiers for naps and nights only. Your baby has started to babble and make noises with their mouth, and keeping a pacifier in their mouths constantly prevents this much-needed verbalization practice. For more information about pacifiers, please see Months 1 and 2.

## Pacifiers and Sleep

Gentle Sleep Coach Heather Irvine, CLEC, reminds us that the nature of sleep is evolving this month, and a lot of the tools or actions that used to help your baby fall asleep quickly no longer do. While the pacifier can still be a helpful tool to soothe your baby, the majority of babies at this stage are not able to control the pacifier on their own—which means that if they rely on the pacifier to get back to sleep, their parents have to retrieve it for them every time they awaken at night. As night wakings increase this month, Heather sometimes sees parents having to run in and reinsert the pacifier every hour!

If you're finding yourself in this situation, Heather suggests several options. One is to make it easier for your baby to reinsert the pacifier on their own. You can use a "pacifier-holding" product: a small stuffy or lovey attached to the pacifier that may help your baby rake it toward their mouth by themselves. You can even try putting one pacifier in each hand to give them multiple options if they wake.

The second option is to wean your baby from their pacifier and replace it with an alternative form of soothing. At this stage, most babies are able to get their hands into their mouth, and if they really want to suck on something, they might even suck on their own tongue and lips. Heather suggests encouraging them to practice using their hands during the day, so that this becomes a workable option for them. Additionally, if they are fussy during the day, you can try waiting to give them their pacifier (for up to 15 minutes) and see if they find an alternative to suck on.

Heather reminds parents that while pacifiers are one of the six recommendations for SIDS reduction, even the AAP recommends pacifier use only at the onset of sleep; there is no need to "replug" your baby after they have fallen asleep. Many babies never take a pacifier in the first place, and their parents rely on the other five recommendations to keep them safe, so it's not necessary to retain the pacifier only for this purpose (please see Before Birth for more on SIDS).

## Pacifier Weaning

Some babies, particularly those who exhibited colic or reflux, are really attached to sucking on something and might find it difficult to self-soothe any other way. This is the earliest age that your baby is able to begin to self-regulate, so they may not be ready to do this on their own. In this case, you may want them to keep using the pacifier (in which case you might need to replug their pacifier at night or use a pacifier-holding product).

If you're looking to wean, we recommend coming up with a solid sleep coaching plan (more on this in the Sleep section) and starting at bedtime after your regular routine. A few options:

- ✫ You can let your baby suck on the pacifier as they fall asleep and then remove it *before* they are completely asleep. You can then pat and shush them to see if they will continue the process of going to sleep without the pacifier.
- ✫ If your baby is particularly attached to the pacifier, you may find that you can get them used to going to sleep without it by starting with 2 minutes of patting and shushing before giving them the pacifier for the night, and then increasing the duration by 2 minutes each night, to see if they will go to sleep without it.
- ✫ If your baby is particularly upset, you can pick them up and rock them to sleep.
- ✫ If you find that this process isn't working at bedtime, Heather recommends trying it during the first nap of the day instead.

With a plan, we see many babies weaned from the pacifier within 2 or 3 days. If you're finding that your baby is particularly upset when you try to put them to sleep without the pacifier but you want to stick with it, you can slow this process down, stretching it over the course of a few weeks. Or, if you are uncomfortable with the amount of crying at this time, you can just halt the process and try it again in a few weeks.

## *Your Baby's Blossoming Self-Soothing Skills*

Up to this point, you've provided soothing to your baby so that they can understand the difference between being regulated and dysregulated. Around this age, your baby becomes capable of very basic self-soothing. They may not be able to completely calm themselves down yet, but they are experimenting and may even be able to put themselves back to sleep using their new skills. Heather shares that babies at this age who figure out how to self-soothe can remember that they have the ability to soothe themselves and also how to repeat the action that helped them do so.

You can start to watch for signs of self-soothing as early as 4 months. Examples include:

- ☆   Rolling.
- ☆   Kicking.
- ☆   Raising and dropping their legs.
- ☆   Squeezing their legs together.
- ☆   Rubbing their head back and forth on a surface.
- ☆   Using a small attachment object.
- ☆   Sucking on their hands.

---

### Reminder: If Your Baby Has Started Rolling, They Can No Longer Be Swaddled

You want your baby to learn to roll, but once they do, it means that swaddling is no longer an option for soothing. If your baby rolls onto their stomach, they will need their arms free to roll to their back again. (At this stage, it is highly likely that your baby has learned to roll one way but not the other.) Check out our suggestions in Month 3 (page 188) for how to wean your baby from the swaddle.

---

While you might be able to see these new self-soothing skills during the day, your baby will also begin to apply them to the "going to sleep" process. This is great news, since sleeping longer stretches at night is dependent upon your baby's ability to soothe themselves back to sleep when they wake. We'll talk about this in more detail later in the chapter.

## SOAR for Soothing

As you learned previously in this chapter, what worked last month to soothe your baby might not work this month, given the developmental changes they're experiencing. You may have to work even harder to be your baby's detective.

When they start to get fussy and your usual soothing techniques don't calm them, take a step back and follow the SOAR process. Keep in mind that even though they might be fussier right now due to the 4-month regression, they are learning new skills this month (like moving their hands to the middle of their body, sucking their hands and fingers, and rolling) that will soon help them better soothe themselves when they get upset. In the meantime, you can view these skills as another way your baby can ask for what they want and need.

Your baby will move through this fussy period. Hang in there!

---

### Stay Off the Roller Coaster

When my eldest daughter entered middle school, the guidance counselor, speaking to a room of parents, told us that our children were going to be on an emotional roller coaster for the next few years. Our job was to not get on the roller coaster with them . . . or if we did (as I sometimes found myself doing), to get off as soon as possible!

This is great advice for weathering your baby's big developmental changes, too. During the fourth month, they are riding a roller coaster of new sensations and frustrations. You want to stay calm, try not to panic, and not jump on the roller coaster with them.

## Soothing Challenges

Most of what you'll be dealing with on the soothing front this month has to do with your baby's changing preferences when it comes to soothing techniques. Something that easily did the trick in the past might not work this month. Just keep experimenting until you find something that does!

### Colic versus GERD

Was your baby fussy and difficult to soothe in previous months, and you labeled this fussiness "colic"? If they are still exhibiting excessive fussiness, check with your pediatrician to rule out GERD or other digestive upsets. Check out Months 2 and 3 for symptoms and soothing solutions. You'll want to get your pediatrician involved as well and also rule out food sensitivities and allergies.

### Teething

If your baby is particularly fussy as you try to calm them for sleep, you may want to determine if they are teething (so you know how to soothe them!). If you think your baby is teething, you can wash your hands and push your finger on their lower front gums—if they cry out, you'll know you have a teether!

Most babies begin to get their primary teeth after the age of 4 months—usually between 6 and 9 months.[111] (Fun fact: If both parents got their teeth early, then the baby is likely to as well!) But the process of teething starts earlier, between ages 3 and 6 months. You may see your baby begin to drool at this time, because teething produces a lot of saliva and they don't yet have the swallowing reflex to take care of it.

As your baby's first teeth start to pop through their lower gum, the area starts to swell, and sucking can make swollen gums feel even worse.[112] This means that if your usual "go-to" for soothing is a pacifier or nursing, these might not currently help.

Instead, Gentle Sleep Coach Gabriela Zepeda, MD, recommends encouraging your baby to chew on textured silicone toothbrushes that are easy to grab—have your baby hold them close to the top, so they don't choke. Holistic pediatrician Ana-Maria Temple recommends offering your baby frozen cubes of breastmilk or formula in a mesh teething bag. (Note: These soothing techniques are for daytime soothing only.)

# TEMPERAMENT

Most temperament research suggests that we can't begin to see our baby's temperament until about 4 months of age. But I've talked to many parents who say they could tell their baby's temperament in the delivery room! That's why I've been teaching you about it since the very beginning. If you feel as if you haven't yet seen your baby's temperament emerge, however, it is likely that you will start seeing it now. And if you have seen it in the past, you are probably now seeing it even more clearly.

As you know, understanding your child's temperament helps you know how to soothe them; what helps one baby in their fourth month might not help *your* baby in their fourth month. But it will also help you know when, and how slow, to sleep coach. By paying attention to your baby's temperament, you'll be able to set realistic goals and select the best sleep strategies from the Transitioning from Sleep Shaping to Sleep Coaching section to support the overall success of your sleep coaching plan.

## The Three Baby Temperaments

The landmark study from 1956 that I introduced in Before Birth—the one that identified the nine basic temperament characteristics—also identified three distinct categories that babies tend to fall under. The study found that most babies can be described as one of the following:[113]

### The Easy or Flexible Baby (most babies fall into this category—around 40 percent)

- ✰ Easygoing and adaptable.
- ✰ Adjusts easily to new situations.
- ✰ Quickly adjusts to routines.
- ✰ Regular sleeping and eating patterns.
- ✰ Easy to calm.
- ✰ Social, cheerful, and in a pleasant mood most of the time.

### The Slow-to-Warm or Shy/Cautious Baby
### (15 percent of babies)

✩	Sensitive, cautious, and shy.

✩	May be difficult to soothe and care for at first but becomes easier over time.

✩	Prefers order and predictability.

✩	Thoughtful.

✩	Sensitive to new experiences.

✩	Needs more transition time to move comfortably between activities.

### The Active/Fussy or Difficult Baby
### (what I call *alert*—10 percent of babies)

✩	Slow to adjust and adapt to change.

✩	Intense, demanding, and moody most of the time.

✩	Unpredictable and irregular feeding and sleeping patterns.

✩	Difficulty with new places, situations, and people.

✩	Intense reactions—willful, obstinate, needs *their* way!

✩	Supersensitive and easily frustrated.

✩	Extremely active and physical.

✩	Needs constant attention.

✩	Determined and resourceful.

**Easy babies** typically do well with most sleep strategies because they are flexible and quick to adapt to new routines. You can usually move through the sleep coaching process without too many hiccups.

**Slow-to-warm babies** need more time to adapt to changes and transition into new routines. You may need to slow down the sleep coaching process for them and initially offer more soothing as you go along. For instance, your baby may need a pre-bed routine that is longer and slower than your friend's baby. Results might seem to come a little bit slower than with easy babies, too. You may first see small changes in their sleep patterns within 3 or 4 days, instead of just 1 or 2.

**Active/fussy (alert) babies** need a lot more soothing and will move even more slowly through changes and new routines. Often, I'll start parents of these babies with the simple step of committing to a regulated bedtime. Even with great effort on their part, they may find improvement to their baby's sleep emerges very slowly.

Eventually, when they get to sleep coaching, it requires a lot of patience on the part of the parents—both because the process is slower and also because the results appear at a slower rate.

Alert babies do *not* do well with anything close to the "cry it out" method. They are easily dysregulated and difficult to calm down. These babies are often more persistent and will cry longer, trying to hold out until they get what they want (namely, an easier, more comfortable way to fall asleep, like nursing or in your arms). These babies can sometimes even develop an aversion to their own crib if not well soothed. So reacting quickly with soothing is imperative. You ideally want to calm your baby and their environment before putting them into their crib, because the calmer they are throughout the process, the easier it will be for them to learn how to self-soothe and go to sleep on their own.

*Does your baby take a long time to get used to changes?*
You may need to take gradual steps.

*Is your baby very sensitive or clingy?*
They may need extra help feeling confident at bedtime and comfortable with their crib and room first.

*Is your baby extra alert, social, or curious? Does your baby show intense reactions? Is your baby highly distractible when nursing or feeding?*
They may not do well with a face-to-face technique, and may need extra help to quiet their busy mind, including a quiet and dark room and a consistent pre-sleep routine.

*Is your baby fairly easygoing?*
They will likely do well with any technique—though we are partial to a gentle one regardless.

*Is your baby very active?*
They may be very wiggly and futz about in the crib more before falling asleep. They may also need more wind-down time before bed, and enjoy a deep-pressure massage. Younger babies may be easier to put down asleep or very drowsy.

*Is your baby slow to warm up to new situations, or pull back when faced with new people?*

They may need a longer bedtime routine or to have the last steps completed in their room to give them time to get used to the idea of falling asleep.

*Is your baby very persistent, easily remaining focused on a task or learning a new skill?*

You may see that they continue to practice new skills such as rolling, or later crawling or sitting, in their sleep, causing more frequent night wakings. Offering lots of opportunities to practice in the daytime will help.

*Do changes cause your baby to get upset or clingy, or to protest?*

They may need to be nursed or comforted for a long time before they can settle at night. These babies especially benefit from a calming and predictable bedtime routine and may cry when they wake if their environment or location has changed.

*Is your baby very sensitive to sounds, textures, and lights?*

You will need to read their cues to determine what makes things better and what makes things worse. Their environment must be just right in order for them to fall asleep and stay asleep. Also note that more sensitive babies may have more disturbed sleep when teething.

## When to Sleep Coach Alert Babies

Gentle Sleep Coach Macall Gordon is often asked why parents of alert babies often wait to sleep coach until 6 months. As you may remember, Macall refers to alert babies as "live wires." She says, "By waiting until your live wire has more skills in their toolbox and sleep development is on your side, you have a better chance of really having some traction with working on sleep."

If you have an alert baby, you may want to bookmark the sleep coaching steps we outline for a later time!

*Is your baby very sensitive to your mood?*

Make sure you calm yourself before bedtime so you can pass that calm onto your baby. They will pick up on your relaxed and positive attitude and get the message from you that it is safe to sleep.

 ## GETTING YOU AND YOUR BABY TO SLEEP

You had the schedule down. Your baby was *finally* sleeping more . . . and then, wham! Suddenly they are not.

What else can you do to support them (and yourself) through the 4-month sleep regression? And what can you do afterward, to get your baby's sleep back on track?

### Sleep Needs in Healthy Full-Term Babies

The typical sleep average for your baby in this fourth month is **10 to 11 hours at night and 4 or 5 hours during the day, spread out over three or four naps (or more, if their naps are short).**

---

### A Refresher on Wakeful Windows

A wakeful window is the length of time your baby can comfortably be awake before they get fussy. But remember, the wakeful window length we give each month is just an average. You'll still want to watch your baby for sleepy cues (the ones that happen before they begin to fuss) in case they get tired earlier, to prevent them from getting overtired and having more trouble falling asleep.

At this age, your baby's wakeful window length is a maximum of 2 hours, based on their current development. Babies who are taking shorter naps may have a shorter wakeful window. It's okay if your baby is taking shorter naps—just try to get more naps in each a day, so they are rested come bedtime.

---

## Getting through the 4-Month Sleep Regression

You learned about the 4-month sleep regression in the Development section of this chapter. While all developmental leaps can contribute to disrupted sleep, this one is particularly disruptive because the development itself is related to sleep. Your baby's sleep cycle is changing in a way that makes it more difficult for them to stay asleep.

While some babies breeze through this period of neurological and physical development, others find their sleep particularly disrupted and become extra fussy. The most important thing to remember this month is that these are very normal reactions to the developmental changes your baby is experiencing. The expectations you have for your little one's sleep may have to be temporarily thrown out the window.

This is a good time to observe your baby and give them the space (without leaving them completely) to figure out what may soothe them for sleep. It's normal for their needs to change. Soothing routines like rocking might no longer work. Often parents will try to do too much in a panic to try to soothe their baby as their preferences are changing, and this can make things worse. Your baby may need a little less of one thing or something completely different—or both! They still need your assistance to help them regulate, but pulling back a bit can help you and them find out what is working for them and what is not helpful.

Even though sleep itself is the "problem," when it comes to the 4-month sleep regression, there are still a few things you can do to support your baby through this time.

First, we recommend that you go back and review all of the Baby-Led Sleep Shaping steps we've recommended so far. Many of them will still work well to help keep your baby's sleep from getting completely off track.

Second, you can add extra feedings or extra soothing to your routines during this time. Don't worry about creating "bad habits" with these additions! We will help you get back on track once your baby is through the regression.

## *Making Sure Wake-Up and Bedtime Are Regulated*

When adults need help with their sleep, the first recommendation they are given is to regulate their bedtime and their wake time, because this helps solidify their circadian rhythm. This works for babies as well!

As parents struggle with their baby's sleep disruption this month, I find that they sometimes forget to adhere to the sleep shaping elements that they previously put in place. For example, they feed their baby when they wake around 6 AM and then put them back to sleep, forgetting that this is their usual wake-up time. When parents regulate their baby's wake-up time, following their baby's natural rhythm, they find that nighttime sleep gets more organized.

At this stage:

- ✩    Your baby's wake time should be between 6 and 7:30 AM.
- ✩    Your baby's bedtime should be between 6:30 and 8 PM.

For more on regulating your baby's wake time, please see Month 2.

---

### Am I Creating "Bad" Habits?

The 4-month sleep regression is draining for everyone, including your baby.

It's not surprising that in your attempts to get your baby to sleep, you may have felt that you created a few so-called "bad" habits. You may be relying on methods that work for now but that you definitely do not want to be used for the next couple of years.

You know what? That's okay! Just know you can easily change these things once your baby is through this milestone and is more capable of self-soothing. Don't worry about creating any "bad" habits. Habits can be changed.

# THE ELEMENTS OF BABY-LED SLEEP SHAPING (MONTH 3 AND BEYOND)

**① CREATE A SLEEP-FRIENDLY ENVIRONMENT**
- Room-darkening shades.
- Soothing colors.
- White noise.

**② CREATE DAILY ROUTINES**
- At bedtime, use your consistent, soothing routine. Do this in your baby's nursery if you plan to eventually transition them there, even if you are currently room sharing.
- Create a shorter pre-nap version of your pre-bed routine.

**③ PREVENT OVERSTIMULATION (FOLLOW THE 3 PM RULE)**

**④ DON'T LET YOUR BABY SLEEP THROUGH A DAYTIME FEEDING (OVER 3 HOURS)**
Have your baby's last nap end 1 to 1½ hours before their bedtime.

**⑤ SUPPORT YOUR BABY'S BUDDING CIRCADIAN RHYTHMS**
- Watch their windows of wakefulness.
- Dim lights at night.
- Expose them to sunshine in the morning.

**⑥ REGULATE YOUR BABY'S WAKE-UP**
For example, wake them for the day at 7:30 AM.

**⑦ REGULATE YOUR BABY'S BEDTIME**
Note the time that your baby usually goes to sleep at night and set that time as their bedtime.

**⑧ FOCUS ON CREATING ONE LONGER STRETCH OF SLEEP AT NIGHT**
Try a dream feed to see if it helps (see page 143).

**⑨ FILL YOUR BABY'S DAYTIME SLEEP TANK**
- Help them get naps any way you can: rocking, holding, pushing them in the stroller.
- Watch for their sleepy cues and avoid letting them get overtired.

**⑩ BEGIN TO MOVE BEDTIME EARLIER**
Each night, move your baby's bedtime earlier by 15 minutes until you are putting them down in their crib between 7 and 8 PM. Bedtime should be no more than 2 hours after their last nap.

## Napping

Your goal for this month is to fill your baby's daytime sleep tank any way you can so that even if they wake a lot at night during this regression, they are still getting enough sleep in each 24-hour period. This means you can let your baby sleep on a walk in the stroller, in a sling while you're wearing them, or in a safe swing.

You may find that getting them down for naps is also challenging, and that they have trouble staying asleep for them. Because of the neurological development your baby is experiencing, they are sleeping a bit lighter during the day as well.[114] Hang tight! Their naps will get easier in the near future.

## Once You've Made It through the Regression

Is your baby starting to sleep better again? Do you see that long stretch of sleep reemerging at the beginning of the night? Does your baby seem less clingy and fussy? Congratulations—you've made it through the 4-month sleep regression!

During the regression, we encouraged you to double down on the Baby-Led Sleep Shaping elements we had taught you (see page 218). We know, however, that you may have deviated from these in favor of getting your baby sleep however you could.

As you come out of the regression, your first step is to go back and make sure that **each of the Baby-Led Sleep Shaping elements is in place**. Getting back to a regular rhythm during both day and night will not only help your baby's sleep but also let you assess if they are ready for Baby-Led Sleep Coaching.

### Readjusting Your Baby's Internal Clock

Now that you are on the other side of the 4-month sleep regression, you may start to see your baby's routines reestablish and their sleeping and feeding schedules get back on track. To help encourage this, expose your baby to lots of natural light during the day. Take them for walks, open the windows, or (if it's warm enough) have some tummy time on a blanket outside. Just 30 minutes in the morning and afternoon will help readjust their internal clock, especially if their sleep was particularly disrupted. For more on supporting your baby's circadian rhythm, please see Month 3.

## Reducing Night Feeds

During the 4-month sleep regression, you may have added a dream feed, or your baby may have awoken more often to be fed and now have become used to these additional nightly feedings. Now, you may be looking to wean your baby of these additional feedings.

After reestablishing any gentle sleep shaping elements that fell by the wayside during the regression, start by making sure that your baby's feeding is going well during the day. Then, you can turn your attention to weaning feedings at night.

You'll want to do this gradually. One option to reduce the number of ounces you put in their bottle or the number of minutes your baby is at the breast slowly, over the course of a few nights.

For example, Gentle Sleep Coach Heather Irvine, CLEC, recommends that if your baby is taking a dream feed before midnight, you can reduce that dream feed by 1 to 2 minutes each night if breastfeeding, or by ½ to 1 ounce if bottle-feeding, over the course of a week or so. Once your baby gets down to a 2-minute nursing session or only 2 ounces in the bottle, you can wean them altogether.

---

### ☁ Sleep Lady Tip ☁

Talk with your doctor (and lactation consultant, if you are breastfeeding) to find out what night feedings should look like for your baby. How many feedings does your baby need given their age, weight, growth, health, and how often or well they are feeding during the day? Can they be weaned?

---

## Evaluate Your Baby's Readiness for Sleep Coaching

Now that the regression has passed, it's tempting to want to start sleep coaching right away. But while some babies may be ready for sleep coaching by 4 to 5 months of age, my Gentle Sleep Team has found that, generally, waiting until 6 months will bring you results faster and cause you less frustration.

I don't recommend sleep coaching until after a baby has gone through the 4-month sleep regression, at a minimum. The absolute best time to teach your baby positive long-term sleep habits is after their brain and central nervous system have matured, and this usually takes 6 months. Many other experts agree that 6 to 8 months is the perfect window to work gently with your baby to teach them healthy sleep habits and self-soothing skills. Based on our readiness checklist and your gut, you can determine when your baby is ready. It's always okay to wait.

---

## Early Sleep Coaching

As you learned in Start Here, babies who are sleep coached too early will take much longer to learn the skills and are more likely to cry longer and harder without showing signs of self-soothing. It is always better for your baby if you wait until they are developmentally capable of learning self-soothing skills.

---

Gentle Sleep Coach Macall Gordon, MA, helps parents understand why we wait on sleep coaching by comparing it to other areas of parenting. Parents worry that helping their baby fall asleep at this age will give them future sleep issues. But do we refuse to dress our children for fear that they won't ever be able to dress themselves? Refuse to spoon-feed an infant for fear that they'll never be able to use a spoon themselves? No!

Macall shares a few other reasons parents often wait to sleep coach until 6 months. Before, "sleep patterns have been fairly fluid and variable. By 6 months, however, sleep shifts into a new level of organization. All of those short, frequent naps consolidate into three predictable longer naps. Babies are also able to go longer without feeds and are able to do more of the work of going to sleep, with a little less help than before. Six months is also when many parents are ready to move their baby's crib out of their room."

## The Case against Cry It Out

If you've read Start Here, you know how I feel about the "cry it out" method. When parents ask me about this method, I remind them where babies are developmentally at this age. Babies are incapable of self-soothing themselves out of intense crying. And on top of that, intense crying means that they are dysregulated and not in a state to learn something new.

As Macall says, "The notion that learning is taking place when babies are hysterical just doesn't make sense. We want to nudge children into better patterns, not throw them into the deep end. Stepping in to help them manage big feelings is in our parent job description. It's no different with sleep."

Baby-Led Sleep Shaping and Coaching are effective because the parent is gently nudging their baby into new patterns when the baby is ready—following the baby's lead, rather than pushing them to do something that is outside their current capabilities.

### BABY-LED SLEEP COACHING READINESS CHECKLIST

If you want to know if your baby is ready for Baby-Led Sleep Coaching—the next step in their learning—take a look at the following checklist. But please know that there is nothing wrong with your baby if they are not yet ready. It's also okay to think your baby is ready, find that they are not, and wait another month or so to try again.

Your baby may be ready for sleep coaching if:

- ✩ Your baby is at least 4½ months old and through the 4-month sleep regression.
- ✩ You are beginning to see a pattern in your sleep logs, including:
  - A regular wake time in the morning—between 6:30 and 7:30 AM.
  - A consistent bedtime between 6:30 and 7:30 PM.
  - One long stretch at night. (It's okay if they don't have this now, as long as they used to before the regression.)

✴ You have a relaxing, soothing, and consistent bedtime routine.

✴ Your baby goes down and stays down easily for naps and gets the amount of sleep during the day that is expected for their age (no matter how you get them to sleep and even if they're still taking lots of short naps).

✴ Your baby's doctor has stated that it's okay for your baby to feed only one to two times overnight and has given you the green light to start gentle sleep coaching.

✴ Your baby is getting enough to eat during the day (according to their age).

✴ Any feeding and health challenges (like reflux or allergies) either have been treated or are well managed.

✴ Your baby's growth is on target.

✴ You have had some success with sleep shaping tips and either the Switch-eroo or Jiggle and Soothe at bedtime.

✴ All family members and other caregivers involved are on board.

✴ You are prepared to stop coaching if it becomes difficult or your baby gets too frustrated.

If you feel that most of these statements describe you and your little one, you may choose to try gentle Baby-Led Sleep Coaching. However, I'd suggest you wait a few more weeks to start sleep coaching if any of the following are true:

✴ Your baby still wakes frequently and takes full feedings at night.

✴ Your baby has had a drastic change in their sleep pattern due to the 4-month sleep regression and you haven't gotten back on track yet.

✴ You suspect that your baby is still in the throes of the 4-month sleep regression.

✴ Your baby is starting some form of childcare for the first time.

✴ You need your baby to take a bottle but your baby is struggling to do so.

✴ Reflux or feeding challenges are still present.

✴ Your baby has a more alert and/or sensitive temperament, and you know in your heart you need to wait and stick with sleep shaping for now.

✴ You are not mentally or emotionally ready to sleep coach (that's okay!).

## Transitioning from Sleep Shaping to Sleep Coaching

As a reminder, *sleep shaping* is laying the foundation for sleep by setting up a gentle structure for the day and night; it's about establishing the timing of sleep, following soothing routines, and creating a sleep-inducing environment. *Sleep coaching* is using strategies designed to teach a baby to fall asleep and go back to sleep independently—which often includes strategies that support longer stretches at night without feeding. Sleep coaching includes gently weaning a baby off sleep crutches (negative sleep associations) such as pacifiers, rocking to sleep, nursing or bottling-feeding to sleep—anything a baby needs to go to sleep and back to sleep that requires someone or something other than themselves.

All of the sleep methods we teach exist on a continuum that starts with the gentle foundation of Baby-Led Sleep Shaping and moves on to methods that fit under the definition of sleep coaching. We also have a few new techniques that we consider bridges to the world of sleep coaching: the *Super Slow Shuffle* and *Jiggle and Soothe 2.0*. While we define them as sleep coaching, they share quite a bit with sleep shaping and are a gentle way to move from one to the next.

These gentle sleep coaching methods build on the techniques you learned last chapter: the Jiggle and Soothe and the Switcheroo:

1. The *Super Slow Shuffle* uses the basic moves from the Switcheroo to slowly change your baby's sleep associations to being put in their crib and then patted and shushed to sleep (eventually doing the first part more quickly and patting and shushing less).
2. With the *Jiggle and Soothe 2.0*, you will wake your little one a bit more than in the original Jiggle and Soothe and experiment with patting and shushing them to sleep a bit less.

Once you are confident that your baby has a strong sleep shaping foundation, you can try one of these two bridge techniques at bedtime after a great day of naps (any way you can get them!). We'll walk you through each of these techniques in depth.

## The Super Slow Shuffle

The Super Slow Shuffle is an option I recommend for alert babies who are past the 4-month sleep regression but might not be ready for sleep coaching. I also suggest this method for parents who tell me that they, themselves, are particularly sensitive. These parents know that there will be some level of crying involved in sleep coaching but feel that it will be best for them to take the process extra slowly in hopes of reducing that crying significantly (because as a general rule, the faster a parent-baby team moves through the sleep coaching process, the more tears there are).

Here are the steps to the Super Slow Shuffle:

1. Wait to start practicing this technique at bedtime first, after a day when you were able to fill your baby's daytime sleep tank, getting them naps any way that you can.

2. At bedtime, follow your soothing, consistent routine. Make sure that this routine is consistent and well established and that bedtime is between 6:30 and 7:30 PM.

3. The first night, you'll start putting your baby to sleep the way that your baby is accustomed to. This might be rocking or nursing (see page 226) to sleep. You're going to start by switching their association with this "going to sleep" position. For example, if you normally rock your baby upright to sleep on your shoulder, instead of completely putting them to sleep in that position, try slowly moving them into a more horizontal position and rocking them to sleep that way.

   Your baby may adjust easily to this switch, or you may need to take this step slowly over several nights. Once they have gotten comfortable with the new position you've chosen, you can move on to the next step.

Note: These next few steps might take several nights—or your baby might adjust quickly in one night. Go at your own pace!

# BABY-LED SLEEP SHAPING AND COACHING™

A gentle approach led by your baby's unique temperament and needs.

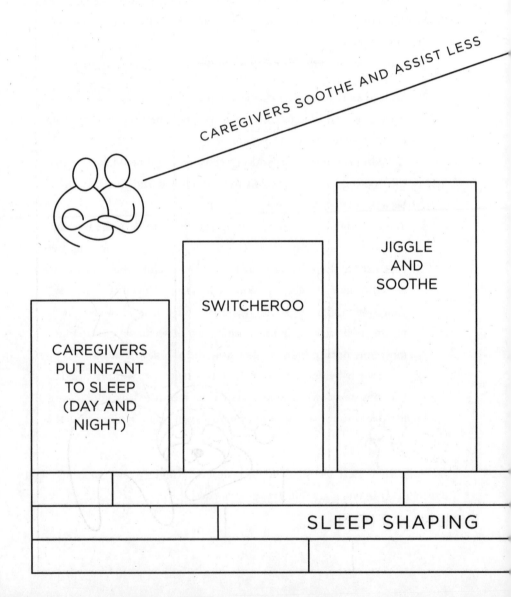

CAREGIVERS SOOTHE AND ASSIST LESS

JIGGLE AND SOOTHE

SWITCHEROO

CAREGIVERS PUT INFANT TO SLEEP (DAY AND NIGHT)

SLEEP SHAPING

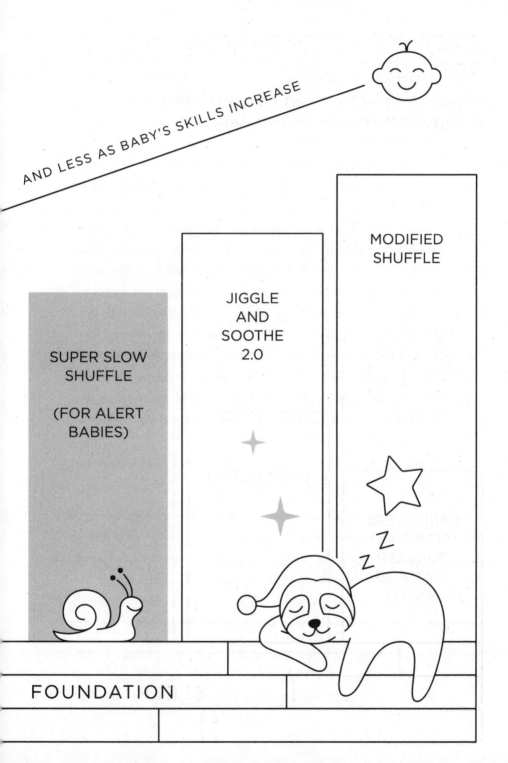

AND LESS AS BABY'S SKILLS INCREASE

MODIFIED
SHUFFLE

JIGGLE
AND
SOOTHE
2.0

SUPER SLOW
SHUFFLE

(FOR ALERT
BABIES)

FOUNDATION

4.  With your baby in their new "going to sleep" position, start to—very slowly, very gently—hold your baby a bit farther from your body, so that you have less bodily contact. You may hold them away with your arms a bit outstretched, or you might move them to your lap, with your arms right next to them for safety. Keep them in this position until they are almost asleep.

5.  Next, carry your baby *slowly* to their crib or sleep space and *very* slowly lower them in, shushing and speaking calmly and softly as you go.

6.  Keep one or both of your arms around them as they lie in the crib. You'll be reaching so far into the crib that it might actually feel like you are *in* it with them. (Believe it or not, I *have* had some parents get into the crib with their babies! You do not need to do this, however.)

7.  Slowly remove your arm(s) or upper body from the crib while patting and shushing your baby. You can hang over the crib and have your face close to your baby if they like it. **This is where you read your baby and follow your intuition. Really let this be a baby-led process! Some babies like a lot of close contact while others are happy with a light hand on them, just letting them know that you are still there.**

8.  Slowly start to stand, continuing to pat them over the railing, as you shush them fully to sleep.

Once your baby is asleep, you may decide to sleep on a mattress in their room for the next several nights so you can respond to them quickly when they wake. You have a few different options for these nighttime wakings. If you feel your baby is adapting well to the new method, you can repeat the Super Slow Shuffle. Or you can simply get them back to sleep any way you can. Try to make the same choice for all wakings, whether they involve a feeding or not, for the rest of the night.

9.  Once your baby is feeling comfortable with these changes (you'll know because they are falling asleep faster and you are feeling more empowered), you can start doing less once they are in their crib and

then eventually less before putting them into the crib. Think of it like a sliding scale where you do less and less as your baby does more. If things are going well, you can try moving through the steps a bit faster to see if your baby has the skills to adjust to the changes at a quicker pace. You can always slow the process back down again if your baby is not ready.

## Jiggle and Soothe 2.0

How did your baby do with the Jiggle and Soothe technique in Month 3? After rousing them slightly, were you able to then pat and shush them back to sleep? If they responded well, I suggest trying the upgraded version of this method as a next step, before moving on to the next level of sleep coaching:

1. Put your baby down to bed already asleep. This means that you can use whatever soothing methods you've been using (feeding, rocking, shushing, patting, etc.) to help your baby get there.

2. Once you lay your baby down in their crib, gently jostle them, **waking your baby a little bit more than you did last month**. They may even look around their sleep space so they know where they are; you can talk to them and tell them where they are as well.

3. Pat and shush your baby back to sleep, just as you did last month. You can practice patting and shushing more intermittently, too! The idea is that you are doing a tiny bit less each night to put them back to sleep. You are following your baby's lead—watching how they respond while offering reassurance as they learn and intervening when they get too upset.

4. If your baby wakes fully or becomes upset, pick them up and comfort them back to sleep.

5. Try the steps again the next night.

Next month, we will help you take your coaching a bit further by teaching you to put your baby in their crib "calm but awake" with the *Modified Shuffle*—if you feel your baby is ready.

Be gentle with yourself! This approach takes patience. Your baby may experience some discomfort even though you are right by their side. If you feel that you are not up for experiencing their frustration at this time, it is okay to wait until you feel that you and your baby are *both* ready.

## Co-Sleeping This Month

If co-sleeping is working for you, please continue to make sure that it is safe, especially if your baby is now able to roll. If you find that it is no longer working, and you'd like to transition your baby out of the family bed, please see the steps I recommend in Month 5.

 Feeling overwhelmed? One of our Gentle Sleep Coaches would love to help you create your sleep plan and support you as you coach your baby through it! Visit FindaSleepCoach.com.

## PMADs

Please make sure that you and your partner are keeping your eyes out for signs of postpartum mood and anxiety disorders. If you see even the slightest sign, check with a trained professional. (If you need help finding one, see PSIDirectory.com.) There is no reason to suffer when there is help out there!

## YOUR SELF-CARE

Yes, you are sleep-deprived! And this month will likely challenge you. But self-care will help you take on this challenge. It can help you calm your own emotions (keep you self-regulated), help you be your baby's detective, and prepare you for the Baby-Led Sleep Coaching in your near future. It can also help keep you from getting so frazzled that communication with your partner completely breaks down!

### Self-Care and Sleep Coaching

If you choose to sleep coach at this time, what can you do to support yourself through the process?

It might seem like you wouldn't want to add more to your life right now. But adding self-care will actually help you be more patient and consistent with sleep coaching. As your baby's sleep coach, you are leading them through the process of learning to self-soothe and put themselves to sleep. How can you do that when you are run-down and dysregulated yourself?

Take a look back at some of the self-care tools we've covered in previous months and add one or two to your schedule:

- ✫ Meditation (page 46).
- ✫ Mindfulness (page 151).
- ✫ Acupuncture (page 114).
- ✫ Supplements.
- ✫ Joy Practice (page 47).
- ✫ Walking meditation (page 189).

### Tongue Fu! for New Parents

If you and your partner are taking on Baby-Led Sleep Coaching, you'll need to make sure that your communication is strong and that you are on the same page.

Plus, discord with our partners can lead to additional stress in our lives (what, more stress?!) and lead us away from the self-regulated state we've worked so hard to attain.

---

### Gatekeeping

Remember, you don't have to do it all! With the additional sleep disruptions this month, it is imperative that you allow your partner and other caregivers to help with soothing and sleep shaping. Don't take it all on yourself and end up experiencing burnout.

---

Communications expert Sam Horn reminds us that "when we're running on empty, what's on the tip of our tongue is almost always a reaction (rather than a thoughtful response), and reactions make things worse." Sam would like us to learn how to hold our tongues, so that we can *respond* instead of *react*, using a communication approach called *Tongue Fu!* Tongue Fu!'s chief aim is to reduce conflict, and it has been taught in organizations around the world, including Intel, Oracle, Nationwide, and NASA.

Sam teaches us how to replace "Words to Lose" (that cause resentment and resistance) with "Words to Use" (that create rapport and respect). Her Tongue Fu! lesson for new parents rests on five main principles:

1. Ban the word *but*. You can replace this "conflict provoking" word with *and*. The word *and* helps you start your sentence by acknowledging what your partner said and then adding to it in a positive way.

   Example: "I know you're tired, *and* I am, too." (See how that makes both of you right?)

2. Stop with the *shoulds*. We've heard about the dangers of Should-Storms and the parenting myths we tell ourselves about what we "should" be able to do, so why would we turn these "shoulds" on our partners? Instead, try replacing *should* with *next time*.

   Example: "*Next time* you're running late, please call so I know what's going on."

3.  *Ordering* is for restaurants, not for couples. Instead of saying *you need to*, try saying *could you please*.

    Example: "*Could you please* pick up diapers at the store on your way home?"

4.  Turn *can'ts* into *cans*. When you're communicating with your partner about what your little one needs, instead of telling them *not* to do something, try sharing that there might be a better time or approach for what they are suggesting.

    Example: "*Can* you take him outside this afternoon instead? It's supposed to be warmer then."

5.  There's always *something* you can do. Instead of believing that everything is out of our control and there is *nothing* we can do, it helps to find at least one thing (no matter how little!) that we *can* do and communicate that.

    Example: "I wish we could make the family reunion, too. There's *something* we can do, though: We can FaceTime during dinner so we can at least be there virtually!"

## NEXT MONTH

We've taught you some sleep shaping techniques, and next month we'll teach you some actual sleep coaching. Remember, there is always *something* you can do to support your little one's sleep—even if your family is still navigating the 4-month sleep regression.

## ONE-PAGE FAST TO SLEEP SUMMARY

**Month 4 Theme:** *Your baby needs to be soothed through the 4-month regression, and you might want to start evaluating sleep coaching readiness.*

### What to Focus on This Month

1.  If you are still in the 4-month regression phase, double down on the sleep shaping elements we taught you in the first 3 months and implement as many as you can.
2.  If you think you are past the 4-month sleep regression and need to get back on track, add back any sleep shaping elements that you may have let go of to make it through the regression (see page 219). If you added additional feedings at night, check out page 220 for more on weaning one or more of these feedings.
3.  If you are back on track post regression, look at the Baby-Led Sleep Coaching Readiness Checklist on page 222 to see if you are ready for sleep coaching.
4.  If your baby is back on track, try the Super Slow Shuffle for an alert baby (page 225) or Jiggle and Soothe 2.0 (page 229).

### What Not to Worry About

Nap coaching and "keeping up with the Joneses' baby"—you and your baby are on your own journey and will be ready for sleep coaching in your own time.

For a printable PDF of this month's FAST to Sleep Summary plus helpful book bonuses, go to SleepLady.com/NewbornSleepGuide.

# Your Baby's Fifth Month

## *16 to 20 Weeks*

> *This month focuses on teaching you the elements of gentle Baby-Led Sleep Coaching for when you and your baby are ready, including how to create a successful sleep coaching plan and various methods you can incorporate into that plan.*

## Parent Spotlight: Joanne
### *Parents of an 18-week-old son, Henry*

Henry was an alert baby from the beginning. Carol and I knew we had our hands full!

He had reflux and eczema, which we spent the first few months getting under control. Then, just as we thought we had everything under control, he went through the 4-month sleep regression. We had to do everything in the book, and then some, to get him first to sleep and then *back* to sleep. Naps went down to 30 minutes max. Any progress we had made before this milestone was lost. We felt hopeless and even found ourselves fighting with each other.

Everyone kept recommending that we either let him "cry it out" or "Ferberize" him. I am sure that works for some babies, but not Henry. We tried one night, and he cried for an hour! Thank goodness we found Kim. She offered us support and gentle options for sleep coaching, and together, we created a game plan. We discussed his reflux and medication dosage with the pediatrician (and didn't add solids even though many people suggested we start them early to improve his sleep and even reflux) due to his sensitive tummy and not wanting to cause unnecessary discomfort while we were sleep coaching.

We focused on night sleep first and did whatever we could with naps in the meantime to get him the day sleep he needed—even if that meant that our nanny held him for naps. With help from his doctor, we determined that Henry still needed one feeding at night, so we built a dream feed into the plan.

Because Henry was so sensitive and seemed to go from zero to 100 in one second flat, we decided to go very slowly. We spent a few nights doing the Switch-eroo at bedtime, switching from nursing to sleep to rocking to sleep. Then when we were all ready, we did the Jiggle and Soothe at bedtime. Eventually, we did the Jiggle and Soothe 2.0, putting him down less drowsy with more intermittent patting. We discovered pretty quickly that it was better not to pat Henry too much—it just seemed to distract him—so we stayed by his crib and intermittently shushed him, instead. He started to suck on his fist at bedtime and put himself to sleep without us doing anything once he was in his crib. It felt like a miracle had happened!

Kim taught us the Modified Shuffle [which you'll learn in this chapter], and we used it to put him back to sleep when he woke in the middle of the night. After a few weeks, we were able to put him right into his crib after his feeding, and he'd fall back to sleep on his own.

After we saw significant progress at night, we focused on the morning nap. He was almost 6 months old, and he *seemed* ready. And he was! Our life has been transformed. Henry is a happy, well-rested, alert baby. He still keeps us on our toes, and we are learning every day!

## MY BABY IS NOT A NEWBORN ANYMORE

Your baby has become a little person with a personality of their own. And now that you have a better understanding of their temperament, you likely have a better understanding of what works and what doesn't work for them in terms of soothing. Their development has increased their skills, and they are more capable of self-soothing. They might even be ready for sleep coaching!

You may still be working on getting your baby back on track after the 4-month sleep regression. Please don't worry! If you need help getting back on track using sleep-shaping techniques, you can flip back to the suggestions in Month 4.

## DEVELOPMENT

In the fifth month, your baby begins to understand where objects are in relationship to other objects. They now notice that an object can be under, on, beside, or inside another object. They become more aware of the distance between themselves and you or other caregivers. This new awareness can spark some stranger anxiety.

New abilities:

- Understanding distance and relationships between objects.
- Playing with their hands and feet.
- Grasping a toy.
- Responding to facial expressions.

Some babies can also:

- Begin to roll over in both directions.
- Mouth objects.
- Turn toward new sounds.
- Make connections between words and actions.
- Recognize their own name.
- Make vowel-consonant sounds such as "baba."

Your baby is starting to understand object permanence. This means that they will start to understand that when you have left the room, you have not disappeared completely—although since object permanence hasn't fully developed, they may still get nervous and fussy when you move out of view, as they have in the past.

They will also start to see the relationship between cause and effect—making the connection that if they cry, you respond. They learn to cry more deliberately to communicate. They also learn that if they drop a toy, their parent will pick it up for them.

Both of these skills—object permanence and understanding cause and effect—can help them feel safer when alone in their sleep space. They are learning that when they lie in their crib and you go to the bathroom, you still exist even if they can't see you. They have also learned to trust that *When I need you and cry out, you will respond.*

Your baby's growing dexterity and ability to rake objects toward themselves with their fingers will, in a few months, turn into the *pincer grasp*: the ability to pinch their index finger and thumb together to pick something up. This will be how they pick up their pacifier and put it back in their mouth when it falls out in the middle of the night. They will also soon be able to smoothly rotate their wrist to put their thumb or a few fingers in their mouth (instead of their whole fist), which some little ones can use to self-soothe.

## Stranger Anxiety

When your baby is a newborn, they do not have a sense of self. Essentially, they think that you and they are one. They smile at the feet and hands that they see waving, without realizing that they belong to them.

As your baby grows and becomes more aware, they gradually begin to figure out that they are their own little person with their own body, emotions, and thoughts. They finally start to understand that you are the ones who care for them, their own parents (exciting!). When this happens, your baby may become anxious when another person tries to hold them (even Grandma). *Stranger anxiety* is a great sign that you and your baby are bonding. Your baby knows the difference between you and a stranger, and they prefer you!

## Stranger Anxiety versus Separation Anxiety

While they may seem similar, *stranger anxiety* and *separation anxiety* are two different things. *Stranger anxiety* may begin as early as the fifth month. Your baby can tell the difference between you and other caregivers, and they prefer you. *Separation anxiety* is when your baby gets fussy and upset when they are away from you at all (no matter who else they are with). It doesn't normally begin to occur until around 6 or 7 months and tends to come and go in waves.

## *Supporting Development*

As you know, being able to roll both ways (back to belly and belly to back) is a great self-soothing tool to add to your baby's basket—and the best way to move them toward rolling, if they haven't yet mastered it, is plenty of tummy time.

### Tummy Time

In month 5, your baby can handle **up to 2 hours of tummy time a day, broken into several sessions**. As always, pick times when your baby is alert, aware, and social—and not right after feeding so they are less likely to spit up.

### Teaching Rolling during Tummy Time

Looking for motivation to make teaching your baby to roll both ways a priority? If they can roll only one way and become uncomfortable on their stomach (or if you are concerned), you may regularly have to go in at night to "flip the pancake," as I call it, to move them from their front to their back because they are not yet able to do it on their own.

There are several things you can do during tummy time to help your baby learn:

### Rolling Front to Back

When your baby is on their tummy, and they pull one of their legs up under them like a little frog, you can lift their same side arm and help them push off against the ground. You can then give them positive verbal feedback ("Yay!"), so they understand that they have done something important.

### Rolling Back to Front

When your baby is on their back, try showing them a toy by holding it up near their face. Then move the toy to the floor by their side and slide it a few inches away to encourage them to reach for it. As they do, they might work hard enough to roll over on their side toward the toy.

Once your baby seems to be mastering rolling over both ways during the day, I suggest you no longer "flip the pancake" when they roll over at night because they are now capable of moving themselves if they find themselves in an uncomfortable position. (The AAP considers it safe to allow babies at this age to remain on their stomachs if they roll over at night.) Instead, if they wake in the night upset after having rolled, I suggest going into their sleep space and assisting them in rolling without completely doing it for them. Each night do less and less as they master the process on their own.

If you haven't already, you'll need to stop swaddling completely at this time. This is both for safety and to allow them to exercise their new skills and move further down the path to self-soothing.

 FEEDING

If you're moving into the sleep coaching phase, make sure that your baby is getting the recommended daily intake of breastmilk or formula for their age. That way, your baby won't be waking additional times at night to feed because they are not getting enough nutrition during the day.

## Feeding at This Age

On average, babies **feed every 3 to 4 hours during the day**. A good number of babies this age still wake for one feeding at night and a few even wake for two. By

6 months, your baby will consume 6 to 8 ounces (180–240ml) at each of four or five feedings in 24 hours.

## Solids

Many experts recommend starting solids at 6 months of age, but new studies suggest that starting as early as 4 months may help reduce the risk of common allergies.[115] Feeding your baby a variety of foods at this age allows their immune system to adapt and helps them tolerate these foods as they grow.

Before starting to offer your baby solids, it is best to talk to your doctor and confirm that your baby:

- ✧ Is able to sit up without support.
- ✧ Is able to maintain great head control when sitting.
- ✧ Has lost the tongue-thrust reflex (so they don't automatically push food out of their mouth).
- ✧ Follows foods with their eyes and shows eagerness and interest.
- ✧ Opens their mouth wide when you offer food on a spoon.

Eating solids is a social and sensory experience for your baby. They eat facing out, versus being nursed or bottle-fed lying down, and get to experiment with new flavors and textures. They also may not do much actual eating at first. For example, you have to wait until their tongue thrust reflex goes away before they really "get" eating solids. And no matter what you do, food will drip down their chin as often as it gets swallowed in the beginning (capture these adorable moments on camera, if you can!).

### Solids and Sleep

Both underfeeding and overfeeding can affect sleep. If your baby is not getting enough to eat during the day, they will wake more to feed at night. If your baby is getting too much to eat, they might wake with tummy troubles. Make sure you're working with your pediatrician if you decide to start solids early.

Please know that you *can* improve night sleep without supplementing with solids, even though other parents or consultants may tell you it is the only way. Read more about the myth about solids and sleep in Month 4.

## Feeding Challenges

As you get ready to sleep coach or take the next step in sleep coaching, it's helpful to make sure that your baby is not experiencing any lingering feeding challenges that might affect sleep, such as reflux or GERD, reverse cycling, or new night feedings added to get through the 4-month sleep regression.

Month 5 will help you address many feeding challenges, and if you need help weaning those additional feedings, we've got more for you in the Sleep section. Here, we'll look at getting back on track after the 4-month sleep regression and what you can do if your baby goes on a feeding strike.

> Remember your feeding log? My team and I recommend continuing this log as you begin sleep coaching so that you can see that your baby is on track with their daily feeding needs, to assure you that feeding challenges aren't negatively affecting sleep coaching.

### Getting Feeding Back on Track

If you are trying to get your baby back on track after the 4-month sleep regression, we suggest looking back at your sleep log to see how long your baby's first nighttime stretch was before the developmental leap. If you added one or more feedings at night and this long stretch is no longer present, you'll want to work on lengthening it before you consider entering the sleep coaching phase. Please take a look at the advice that Gentle Sleep Coach Heather Irvine, CLEC, gives post-4-month sleep regression in last month's Feeding and Sleep sections (page 220).

### Feeding Strikes

Feeding strikes can happen when a baby starts daycare or, if they were exclusively breastfed, is introduced to formula and/or a bottle for the first time. Some babies will go all day without eating, waiting for their parents. Then, of course, they need to eat at night to make up the calories they've lost, causing reverse cycling.

If you find yourself in this situation, take a look at the Feeding Challenges section in Month 3.

## My Baby Started Snacking Night and Day! What Should I Do?

This is a common age for babies to start snacking a lot during the night because they have become very distracted during the day. I recommend feeding in a quiet room and even using white noise if necessary. You may need to feed them more at night temporarily until their daytime feeding distractibility can be tempered.

I had to do this with Carleigh, who hadn't been a distractible feeder in the past but became one in her fifth month. I started to bring her into a quiet room to feed her and keep to what was our usual routine, making sure she was not too hungry but still hungry enough for her feeding.

Please see the Month 3 Feeding section for help with distractible eaters.

 ## ATTACHMENT

As you move from Baby-Led Sleep Shaping to Baby-Led Sleep Coaching (whether that's this month or later on!), you will rely on the trust you have built up and the bond you have forged over the last several months. Keep this trust in mind as you let your baby lead you through the coaching process. Your baby still needs to know that you are close by and will respond if they really need you.

 ## SOOTHING

By now you may feel like you have a decent handle on why your baby cries or fusses (most of the time!) and are using SOAR to help figure out your baby's patterns and temperament and therefore what works and what doesn't work to soothe them. On top of all that, as you have learned, your baby has more self-soothing and communication tools in their toolbox!

## Your Baby's Newfound Self-Soothing Skills

This month your baby may exhibit even more forms of self-soothing that relate to sleep:

- ✩  Turning or rolling away (which they can also use at night to change positions on their own, instead of waking you to help them).
- ✩  Pushing away the bottle or breast when not hungry (which helps you understand what their night feeding needs are at this age).
- ✩  Fussing and crying and rubbing eyes when tired (a clearer cue to help them get to sleep before they become overtired).
- ✩  Thumb or finger sucking (more below!).

These baby steps in communication will help you understand your infant's cues even better.

## Supporting Your Baby with Soothing

Your baby is starting to self-soothe, and you can help them learn self-soothing techniques as well as help remind them of these options when they are upset or fussy. This includes:

- ✩  Encouraging them to roll back over once they have rolled one direction and gotten "stuck."
- ✩  Helping them find their thumb or fingers, if you know that they find sucking particularly soothing.

### Thumb Sucking

I find that some parents have a lot of negative feelings about thumb sucking. Perhaps they have heard horror stories about orthodontist bills down the road—though pediatric dentists have confirmed that a child's need for orthodontic care is related more to their genetics than anything else. However, thumb sucking (or the "hand sandwich," where they put their entire hand in their mouth) can be very helpful because it allows a baby to self-soothe at a young age (you even see ultrasound images of some babies sucking their thumbs in utero).

You may not be able to control if your baby becomes a thumb sucker. There are some benefits, however. If your baby is sucking their thumb, it means that they are self-soothing, which means that something in their world (external environment or even inside them) has made them uncomfortable. Thumb sucking can become a clue to their needs. It may be a sign that they are getting tired and ready for sleep. Or it may be a sign of worry, showing you that they need further soothing to keep them regulated as they try to process and understand a new environment or new people.

## Soothing Challenges

Although your baby has some new self-soothing skills this month, your soothing help is still invaluable, because they are still figuring how to use these skills to regulate themselves.

### Soothing Stranger Anxiety

Remember, stranger anxiety is actually a good sign! It means that your baby is creating a strong bond with you. It can still be difficult to navigate, however.

Here are a few things that you can do to help your baby become comfortable with new visitors and caregivers:

- Add extra soothing. If your baby is soothed by sucking their thumb or fingers, encourage them to do so by bringing their hand to their mouth. Or you may find that your baby naturally starts to suck their thumb during these transitions.
- Offer other soothing objects, like a pacifier or a lovey.
- Be friendly. Your baby is learning social cues from you, so make sure that you demonstrate how much you like and trust this new person before you hand them over.

✿  Don't stress. If your baby has a meltdown while someone else is holding them, don't get upset. Just calmly take them back into your arms to soothe them.

✿  Take extra time. The first time you leave your baby with a new caregiver, take a few extra minutes to play with them and the new caregiver. This is another way of showing your baby that this new person can be trusted.

✿  Create goodbye and reunion routines. Your baby will start to recognize these transitions and anticipate what comes next.

—  Always say goodbye. Your baby may not be able to speak yet, but that doesn't mean they don't understand that you're leaving.

—  Don't linger. After saying goodbye, leave quickly to avoid triggering a meltdown.

✿  Keep trying. It may take your baby a while to adjust to a new person or new environment, so you'll need to be persistent.

In the meantime, you may want to inform family and friends who want to come visit what to expect so they know to be understanding and accommodating and not take it personally!

Eventually your child will move through their anxiety around strangers. It will fade on its own with time, but by doubling down on your bond with them as you continue to expose them to new people and experiences, you can still help them to transition smoothly while it's here.

 ## TEMPERAMENT

Temperament can be an enlightening window into what makes your baby behave the way they do, helping you respond to them in a way that will make life easier, and we are finally at the age when experts all agree that your baby's temperament is truly emerging. You may have recognized your baby as an alert baby several months ago, but now you're really learning the nuances of the associated traits and which ones apply to your child. Perhaps your baby is particularly sensitive but not intense. They may get fussy in a loud room, but their fussiness isn't more intense than other babies' fussiness. Or perhaps your alert baby goes from zero to 100 in what feels like 3 seconds flat when they are hungry, but doesn't seem to mind a dirty diaper.

## Nurturing Your Baby's Unique Nature

Over the years, both scientists and parents have debated the extent of our ability to mold temperament. Research now suggests that 50 percent of temperament is based on nature and 50 percent is based on nurture. When it comes to sleep, I find that nature matters much more. I regularly hear the myth that parents can train their babies to sleep in loud environments. Unfortunately, this is not the case. Either your baby's temperament will allow them to do so (if you are lucky!), or it won't.

You've learned that attachment comes from being properly attuned to your baby and their particular needs. Learning your baby's temperament—their nature—allows you to nurture them as they are instead of trying to fit a square peg into a round hole. Our aim is not to change our babies, but to accept who we have been given . . . even (especially!) if their temperament is not the one we envisioned or wanted. Perhaps your baby doesn't sleep well hiking or camping, but you've learned to work with being closer to home while still feeling like you have an "adult life." You'll continue to learn to love the time with your baby even when they are not who you imagined they'd be.

My alert baby was harder and more interesting to parent. She had more intense tantrums and didn't respond to the same things her older sister had; I had to figure her out. As she got older, she required a different parenting style (and did I mention she was definitely harder to parent?) in that she required me to be more patient, diligent, and consistent in my promises and "rules" or guidelines.

Give your baby the chance to be who they are. You will be rewarded greatly, and so will they!

## Sleep Coaching Alert Babies

You can expect your alert baby to push back against sleep shaping and sleep coaching. When you change familiar patterns, these smart little cookies will let you know that they notice. They will also let you know, loud and clear, that they don't like it. Do what you can to push through. As long as you are present and support-ive, it's okay for them to hate the change. If you can acknowledge their difficulty and just keep going, they will use their powerful brain to pick up on the new pattern—and alert babies love a good pattern.

The worst thing you can do with an alert baby is to commit to a sleep strategy and then when they fuss just give up and do whatever works. If you're inconsistent, your child will not overlook it. If you start out patting and shushing and then end up just feeding them to sleep, for example, they will know that feeding is "on the table" as a possibility and they just have to hold out for it. The next time you try, it can be ten times harder. Set your mind to whatever you are choosing to do and try not to waffle. Remember, you have to stay one step ahead of your alert child. They don't miss a thing!

---

## Alert Babies Are the Ones I See the Most

As I've mentioned, around 75 percent of the clients who come to me have alert babies—because alert babies often have sleep difficulties. They have a harder time shutting the world out to go to sleep and often need *all* of the sleep environment suggestions I make: the consistent pre-sleep routine, quiet, room-darkening shades, regular sleep times, and sleeping in their own sleep space. They are not as adaptable for the first few years and won't easily sleep in the car or in a stroller (or on vacation!).

If you've been blessed with an active, engaged, stubborn child, you also might be particularly sleep-deprived. Please don't despair if you've gotten to this point and your alert baby is still not sleeping well. You may have to implement my Baby-Led Sleep Shaping elements and Baby-Led Sleep Coaching strategies at a slower pace, but there is sleep at the end of the tunnel!

GETTING YOU AND YOUR BABY TO SLEEP

## *Your Baby's Sleep at this Age*

In their fifth month, your baby may be sleeping much longer stretches at night, or even be sleeping through the night (defined as sleeping 6 hours or more in a stretch). While some babies may sleep from dusk until dawn, a good number of babies this age still wake for one feeding, and some even wake for two.

## *Sleep Needs in Healthy Full-Term Babies*

The typical sleep average for your baby in the fifth month is **10 to 12 hours at night** and **3½ to 4 hours during the day, spread out over three or four naps.** Your baby should also be able to stay awake anywhere from 2 to 2¼ hours between naps, depending on nap length.

## *Ready for Sleep Coaching?*

Not all babies are ready for sleep coaching at this stage. I've worked with 8- and 9-month-olds who weren't yet ready for sleep coaching. Sometimes it has to do with the baby's temperament, or a difficult beginning, or an illness that they are getting over. We need to take all these things into account when creating a plan and choosing a start date.

If you are wondering if your baby might be ready for sleep coaching, please take a look at the Baby-Led Sleep Coaching Readiness Checklist on page 222.

> Sleep coaching readiness in premature babies should always be based on their adjusted age, even if they are "caught up" in other areas.

As you prepare to begin sleep coaching, make sure you're taking into account any lingering issues that might affect the success of your plan. Was there a particularly traumatic birth that still requires some recovery for either you or your baby? Are you or your partner feeling guilty about returning to full-time work? Have there been feeding difficulties or any underlying medical concerns? If you answer "yes" to any of these questions, sleep coaching might be a bit more challenging for your family.

I want you to commit only to what you feel comfortable with and can follow through with consistently. Go over your goals and look at your family's schedule. Do you feel like you are particularly sleep-deprived and need to address your baby's sleep sooner rather than later? Do you have the recommended 3 weeks to devote to the process? Or would you feel better waiting?

In the rest of this section, I'll introduce you to some gentle sleep coaching techniques for both bedtime and nap time, and then help you create your personalized Baby-Led Sleep Coaching plan.

> If you don't feel like your baby (or you!) is quite ready for sleep coaching, we encourage you to revisit the sleep shaping sections in Months 3 and 4. If you are feeling great about your baby's sleep shaping foundation, you can try Jiggle and Soothe 2.0 or the Super Slow Shuffle (see the Sleep section of Month 4, page 215) as an interim step ahead of the gentle sleep coaching described in the following pages.

## How Fast "Should" I Sleep Coach?

How quickly you choose to sleep coach will depend on your goals for your baby's sleep (and your own). It will also depend on your baby's temperament (and your own). As you know, the sleep coaching that I recommend is gentle, but changing patterns almost always results in a few tears. I find that when parents speed up the process, the tears tend to increase a bit. **If you are particularly sensitive to your baby's cries, you might want to go slow.**

With alert babies, going too fast can be an issue—but so can going too slow, because your baby can get too comfortable with one stage of the process, making it even more difficult to move on to the next. You'll need to find a nice middle ground, keep evaluating how your baby is doing at your chosen speed, and adjust as needed.

## Your Sleep Log Will Keep You on Track

Remember to keep a sleep and feeding log during your sleep coaching so that you can assess what is working and what is not. It is too difficult to keep all the information you want to remember in your head; the nights in particular will blur together. It will be difficult to see progress . . . and you don't want to miss that! Your log will help you see any patterns, good or bad, as they start to emerge.

I recommend recording the following:

- What time you put your baby down for the night.
- How long it took them to get to sleep.
- What your baby did—for example, fussing, crying (how much and how long), rolling over, trying any soothing behaviors.
- What you did or didn't do—for example, patting, shushing, picking them up to calm them.
- How often your baby woke, what you did at each waking, and how long they were awake.
- The number of night feedings.
- What time you started the day.

You'll also want to log all nap times and lengths and daytime feedings. If you need to determine the source of a sleep coaching challenge later, you can look back and see if the cause might lie in a change in their behavior or activities.

To be clear, it's okay to go *very* slowly if you find that's what is best for your baby. Alert babies often need microsteps in the sleep coaching process. You may feel frustrated that your baby can't move faster. And you may feel like you are the only one moving as slow as a turtle. But trust me, other parents of alert babies are right there with you!

I work with some families at this stage who simply need help committing to a well-regulated routine throughout the day in order to set the stage for sleep coaching in the near future. It's okay to take baby steps. Sometimes, in their excitement to get their baby sleeping, parents bite off more than they can chew. They may decide to address too many aspects of sleep coaching at once when their baby isn't yet ready—leading to more tears and frustration than necessary for both baby and parents. It's also okay to hit pause and come back to sleep coaching when you and your baby are ready.

## Baby-Led Sleep Coaching

When you commit to sleep coaching, you're committing to teaching your baby to learn to fall asleep without parental assistance. I want you to provide your baby with support while remembering that sleep is a learned skill—one that they develop with our reassurance and guidance.

My sleep coaching method for babies this age who are developmentally ready is called the *Modified Shuffle* (which is not the same as the "regular" Sleep Lady Shuffle).

### Introducing the Modified Shuffle

For years, I've taught a method for sleep coaching called the *Sleep Lady Shuffle*. It is a tool that I teach in my book *The Sleep Lady's Good Night, Sleep Tight* to help parents gently support their children, 6 months to 6 years old, as they learn to put themselves to sleep and back to sleep independently. I've created an even gentler version that is more age appropriate for babies under 6 months called the *Modified Shuffle*. It includes many of the same "steps" as the Sleep Lady Shuffle but goes at a slower pace while adding a few new steps and eliminating a few others. (For example, those of you familiar with the Sleep Lady Shuffle will notice that we don't include the "hall in view" step in the Modified Shuffle.)

## THE MODIFIED SHUFFLE, STEP BY STEP

The step-by-step process of the Modified Shuffle allows you to gradually diminish your role in helping your baby fall asleep, giving them the room to figure out how to soothe themselves. The idea is to be their coach, not their crutch.

Think of the Modified Shuffle as a kind of weaning for sleep: You are there providing physical and verbal reassurance while, over the course of a week or two, doing less and less as your baby learns the skill to put themselves to sleep independently. It is the tried-and-true method my coaches and I have been teaching for years to help parents and caregivers teach their young babies to sleep. (For the co-sleeping version, please see page 273.)

1. After a great day of naps (any way you can get them), go through your standard bedtime routine (e.g., diaper change, pjs on, into sleep sack, feeding). After the last step of this soothing routine, turn off the light and turn on your dim night-light (this low light will allow you to safely navigate your baby's room for sleep coaching).

2. Place your baby down in their crib "calm but awake." This means that you have not put them to sleep with nursing, rocking, waking, or patting, and that they are dry, fed, warm enough, loved, and starting to get tired when you put them in their crib.

3. *Nights 1 to 3:* Stay close by (even standing next to the crib) and comfort your baby with touch and verbal reassurance until they fall asleep (patting, gently rocking them back and forth, jiggling, shushing, providing verbal reassurance, or whatever works for you and your baby). This is a time when they might really need us to pick them up and calm them down. I am all for using touch, eye contact, and/or your voice to calm them. You can even pick them up—but once they're calm, put them back in their crib. Don't worry about doing "too much" patting and shushing the first couple of nights. You both may need it, and you can focus on doing less over the next couple of nights.

   *Note:* You may find that your baby seems more upset when you make eye contact or is more visually stimulated in general. For these babies, I suggest parents try patting them through the bars of the crib (versus over the top of the rail) and continuing the "shushing" and vocal calming and seeing if that works. Similarly, some babies don't like a lot of patting but may be comforted by shushing. You can also sit on the floor and offer shushing from there. Experiment with what works for you and your baby.

The goal is to help your baby fall asleep *in their crib*—even if that means your entire upper body is in the crib with them (assuming that seems to help, of course!). Each night, you will gradually reduce your physical reassurance (by standing up rather than bending over the rail and patting less) and use more verbal reassurance. However, it's okay to practice this step for a few nights longer if you have a particularly sensitive baby (just as we suggested with the Super Slow Shuffle).

4. *Nights 4 to 6:* Put your baby in their crib and sit on a chair a few feet away or on the floor nearby, continuing to offer verbal reassurance— for example, shushing or singing. If your baby is particularly fussy, first wait a beat, but then return to the side of the crib to verbally soothe them. If shushing and the sound of your voice doesn't soothe them, you can go back to patting them. A particularly upset baby may need to be picked up to calm down. Once they are calm, you'll want to put them back in their crib and see how little verbal or physical reassurance you can give them before they are calm enough for you to move back to your chair or the nearby spot on the floor. You'll be doing less patting going forward, and therefore this step will be more difficult if you were using a lot of touch during the first 3 nights.

5. *Nights 7 to 9:* Each night, move your chair incrementally farther away from your baby's crib, toward the door, until you no longer feel your baby needs you to stay in the room—because they are easily going to sleep on their own.

## Guidelines for the Modified Shuffle
*(Bookmark this page!)*

These are your "rules of engagement" for standing and sitting by your baby's crib as you do the Modified Shuffle:

- You can **stroke, shush, pat, and rub your baby—but not constantly**. The idea is to do this intermittently so that these actions don't become a new sleep association. You don't want your little one to expect you to "pat and shush" them to sleep every night. (While we did practice this in *sleep shaping*, we have moved on to *sleep coaching* now.)

- You'll want to **carefully manage your level of touch** so that being patted to sleep or falling asleep holding your finger doesn't become just another sleep crutch.

- As you move away from your baby's bed, **reduce the amount or volume of verbal reassurance** so that your baby can learn to sleep without it.

- You can **pick up your baby and soothe them if they become too distraught to fall asleep on their own**, but try not to hold them to sleep. Always try some variation of shushing or patting first to see if that calms them. Throughout the last several months you have become your baby's expert. Use your intuition and past experience to gauge how much frustration your baby can handle with you by their side.

- **It's okay to move at a slower pace** than outlined here. You can spend two extra nights patting them through the bars of the crib. Or you can take an extra night standing at the crib if you think your baby needs it. You can spend more time on any step if you feel that your baby isn't ready to move to the next one (just as we suggested with the Super Slow Shuffle).

# BABY-LED SLEEP SHAPING AND COACHING™

A gentle approach led by your baby's unique temperament and needs.

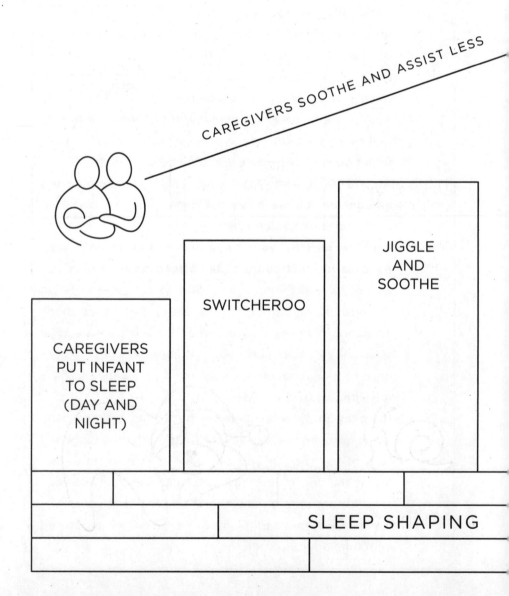

CAREGIVERS SOOTHE AND ASSIST LESS

JIGGLE AND SOOTHE

SWITCHEROO

CAREGIVERS PUT INFANT TO SLEEP (DAY AND NIGHT)

SLEEP SHAPING

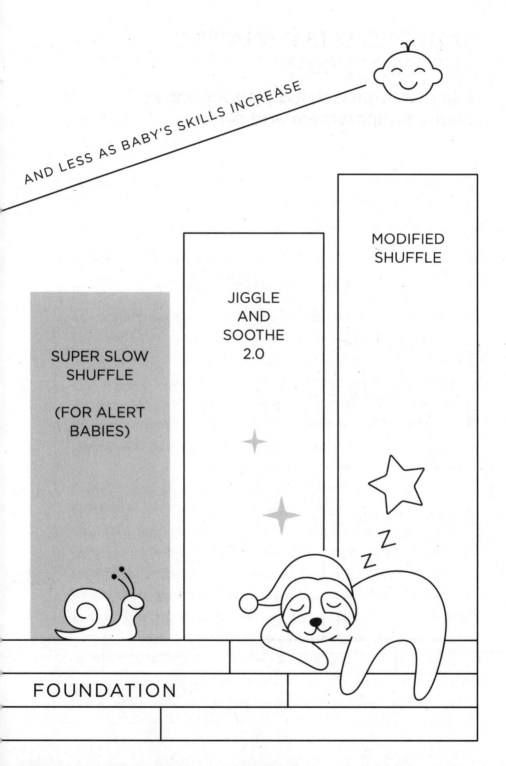

AND LESS AS BABY'S SKILLS INCREASE

MODIFIED
SHUFFLE

JIGGLE
AND
SOOTHE
2.0

SUPER SLOW
SHUFFLE

(FOR ALERT
BABIES)

FOUNDATION

We've broken Baby-Led Sleep Coaching into three phases: coaching at bedtime only, coaching both at bedtime and during night wakings, and nap coaching.

Please choose the phase that is the best match for your baby's temperament and your own. Some parents may decide to skip ahead to Phase 2 and coach their baby both at bedtime and back to sleep when they wake in the night. Others may decide to start with Phase 3 and sleep coach their baby at bedtime, during the night, and for naps.

No matter which phase you choose, always start sleep coaching your baby at bedtime after a day of great naps any way you can get them (and yes, it's okay to use your sleep crutches for those naps!).

## What If My Baby Cries?

I've always found that calling any sleep coaching method "no cry" is a bit of a misnomer and an unfair promise. Yes, there may be fewer tears with a gentler method, and you being right there to comfort your baby as soon as the baby begins to fuss will definitely reduce crying, but that does not mean your baby will not cry *at all* while they are learning a new skill. And the amount and intensity of that crying will depend on temperament, past experience, age, and more.

I recognize how hard it is to listen to your baby cry. I couldn't stand to hear my girls cry either—but I had to remind myself that crying is a normal part of childhood. For those little ones who are nonverbal, crying is how they communicate discomfort, frustration, or even that they just want to be moved to a different position. **Gentle sleep coaching is all about letting your baby sit with a little frustration while you provide support, so that they can successfully learn to sleep on their own.**

The sleep coaching process can be a little stressful for everyone involved, and sometimes babies are simply picking up on their parents' reaction to this new way of going to sleep. If the parent is starting to feel anxious as they work through the sleep coaching steps, this can escalate the baby's reaction as well. If you suspect your baby is distressed because of your reaction, I still don't recommend leaving the room. Instead, I just suggest backing off a bit, or testing sitting on the floor next to the crib and just using your voice, to see if that helps. It may be that a "calmer you" is just what they were craving. If you're feeling anxious, having a different caregiver handle the coaching process might be a good option.

Prolonged, unsupported crying is harmful for babies, so we don't want you to leave your baby to cry unsupported. We want you to be right there reassuring them with patting, shushing, and calming words. Even so, you may be wondering; What is *too much* crying? How long is too long? This is for you to determine. However, if your baby has not had any calm periods in the last 10 to 15 minutes, then please pick them up to calm them. In my experience, a baby who cries (even on and off) for any longer can end up dysregulated—which means that they are both too upset to learn anything new and also more difficult to soothe.

If you decide you are not comfortable with the crying and are beginning to question whether your baby is ready for sleep coaching, or if you realize your baby is particularly sensitive and would benefit from starting later, it is fine to stop and wait until they are older—it will never be too late to sleep coach. If you'd like to continue with sleep coaching but would like an even slower version, we suggest the Super Slow Shuffle in Month 4.

## Phase 1: At Bedtime Only

Because bedtime is often the easiest time for babies to learn the skill of putting themselves to sleep, many parents start sleep coaching first at bedtime only.

During Phase 1, you'll follow these guidelines:

- ☆   Bedtime: Sleep coach following the Modified Shuffle.
- ☆   Night wakings with feeding: Put your baby back to sleep using your usual method before gently transferring them to their crib (often this is nursing or bottle-feeding them until they are asleep).
- ☆   Night wakings with no feeding: Put your baby back to sleep using your usual method before gently transferring them to their crib (for example, rocking or holding them to sleep).
- ☆   Nap time: Put your baby to sleep using your usual method before gently transferring them to their crib.

(Note that you may find that your usual methods stop working during night wakings. If so, you may have to start sleep coaching back to sleep during night wakings as well.)

## How to Start the Modified Shuffle If Your Baby Feeds to Sleep

Many babies feed to sleep (and then back to sleep), but the purpose of Baby-Led Sleep Coaching is to help them learn how to get to sleep without being nursed or bottle-fed. Before starting the Modified Shuffle, switch their association away from feeding to sleep:

1. First start the night with your standard soothing bedtime routine.
2. Then feed them with the light on, both so that they stop associating feeding with falling asleep in the dark and so that you can watch to see when they are done feeding and are about to fall asleep.
3. Before they are asleep, unlatch them or remove the bottle and gently put them in their crib while they are still awake.

You can now start the steps to the Modified Shuffle.

Feeding *back* to sleep is such a common sleep crutch that we've already devoted an entire phase of Baby-Led Sleep Coaching to it. Please refer to Phase 2 for solutions for how to handle night wakings.

## How to Start the Modified Shuffle If Your Baby Is Rocked, Held, or Walked to Sleep

Babies who are accustomed to bouncing or swinging to sleep will particularly miss this movement and activity when you start sleep coaching.

Before starting your pre-bed routine, I suggest walking your baby around the bedroom or rocking them in the bedroom (with the light on) to create a positive association between the room and sleep as a precursor to sleep coaching. After this soothing, go ahead and run through your baby's standard pre-bed routine. Sometimes parents do some rocking and swaying again as they head to turn off the light and put their baby in their crib.

As you lay your baby in their crib "calm but awake," I recommend a very gradual approach where you lean far over into the crib and continue swaying or rocking as you very slowly put them down. This will give your baby more of the rocking and bouncing as they get settled in the crib. Experiment with what works for you and your baby. There is no "one right way" to do this!

You'll want to follow the guidelines for the Modified Shuffle, being very conservative with the "pick up to calm" suggestions. Sometimes babies whose sleep crutch has been holding or rocking will fall asleep in your arms in a minute or two when they are picked up to be calmed, which can train them to cry—something we want to avoid!

If these steps sound like too much all at once, you can follow the steps to the Super Slow Shuffle in Month 4 (page 225). It can take your baby through the process at an even slower rate that might work to help them switch their sleep associations.

## Your Nap Plan in Phase 1

As you'll recall, if your baby naps well during the day, they will sleep better at night. When they get into an overtired state, it is more difficult for them to fall asleep and stay asleep.[116] So, while you are not yet sleep coaching your baby during naps, you still want to pay attention to naps to make sure they are getting enough sleep. Fortunately, changes to your baby's circadian rhythms at this age make this easier!

Your nap plan in Phase 1 is to fill your baby's daytime sleep tank any way you can. This means it's okay to use the swing, the bouncy chair, sleeping in your arms, or even a car ride to get your baby to nap. Let yourself focus on improving nighttime sleep first!

You may find that as your baby masters nighttime sleep, naps get easier as well.

## NAP EXPECTATIONS DURING SLEEP COACHING

Let's take a look at what typical infant naps look like right now:

- ✰ Your baby should be napping **at least three or four times a day, for at least 45 minutes at a time**. (If their naps are shorter—which sometimes happens during sleep coaching—they may need five naps a day). You are working toward **a total of 3½ to 4 hours of daytime sleep**.
- ✰ Naps average between 45 minutes and 2½ hours.
- ✰ Most babies do not transition from three or four naps down to two or three naps until 6 to 8 months. They then transition to two naps after around 9 months if they are sleeping well at night.

It's not uncommon for some babies at this age to be taking several 45-minute naps and then slowly, and on their own, shift to two longer naps and a third shorter nap (which is common for 6- to 8-month-olds).

Because nap lengths still vary at this age, this can, of course, affect their wakeful windows:

- ✰ Shorter nap (45 minutes to 1 hour) = shorter wakeful window (1 to 1½ hours).
- ✰ Longer nap (1 hour or longer) = longer wakeful window (1½ to 2½ hours).

When you look at your sleep and feeding logs, you'll get a sense of your baby's usual wakeful window. You'll probably notice that their first nap of the day typically comes after a shorter wakeful window than usual.

In order to fill your baby's nap tank during sleep coaching, your goal is to get them 3½ to 4 hours of naps a day. This is a range, and the total amount depends both on how much sleep you feel your baby needs in a 24-hour period to be well rested and also on how your baby is sleeping at night. If they are waking more at night, they will be extra tired in the morning, be ready for their first nap a bit earlier, and require more sleep during the day. The number of naps they need will depend on the length of each nap. Don't stress about it! Watch your baby and the clock, and do what you can to get your baby to bedtime without getting overtired.

You'll want to be particularly mindful of your baby's yawns and sleepy cues, which may show up earlier than usual during sleep coaching. That way, you'll be able to start moving them into their next pre-nap routine as soon as you see that they are ready.

Here are my recommendations for getting good daytime sleep:

- ✧ Find the time that your baby often wakes in the morning, and regulate their wake-up at that time going forward (an irregular wake-up confuses their internal clock).

- ✧ Hold off their first nap until after 8 AM to encourage an appropriate wake time. (If they nap before then, often you'll find that you end up with an early rising problem.)

- ✧ For the rest of your baby's naps, watch for sleepy cues and keep an eye on their wakeful windows.

- ✧ Provide an ideal daytime sleep environment (see Before Birth for a reminder).

- ✧ Commit to your pre-nap routine.

## GENTLE NAP EXTENSION STRATEGIES

If your baby regularly takes short naps and still seems tired when they wake, you can try to extend their naps by going into their sleep space 5 minutes before their usual wake-up time and, when they start to rouse a little, soothe them back to sleep, whether by patting them or picking them up to rock them back to sleep. This will help them connect their nap time sleep cycles.

Keep in mind that the last nap of the day is usually the shortest—often just 45 minutes—and that you want your baby to wake from their last nap 2 hours before bedtime.

While sleep coaching can also be used to teach your baby to extend their naps, I strongly suggest waiting to do so until you've successfully sleep coached them through the whole night (see Phase 3 for more).

## Phase 2: Addressing Nighttime Wakings

Once their baby has gotten used to going to sleep in their crib with minimal support (very little shushing or patting), many parents move on to Phase 2: coaching when their baby wakes throughout the night.

### WHEN YOUR BABY WAKES FREQUENTLY AND NEEDS HELP TO GO BACK TO SLEEP

When you begin overnight sleep coaching, you'll want to focus first on night wakings where your baby does not need to nurse or take a bottle.

You and your pediatrician may have determined that even though they wake frequently at night, they do not need to feed each time (or perhaps even at all). They may simply be unable to put themselves back to sleep without being held, rocked, or walked. If this is the case with your baby, you can follow the Modified Shuffle to get them back to sleep each time until 6 AM.

### WHEN YOUR BABY WAKES FREQUENTLY TO FEED: WEANING NIGHT FEEDINGS

Some parents—after determining that their baby is getting enough calories throughout the day—decide that they would like to wean their baby of one or more night feedings.

We recommend reviewing your baby's age, health, and feeding patterns with your pediatrician to determine whether they need to receive calories during the 11-hour nighttime period. If your doctor says that your baby needs to eat during the night, ask them how many feedings they would recommend. You can then plan to gently wean them off the other feedings.

---

Please keep in mind that if your baby is used to eating in the night, it doesn't matter whether they are actually hungry or the night feedings are just a habit—it will still *feel* like hunger. Therefore, we always recommend a gentle, gradual approach to night weaning.

Remember, it is perfectly normal for a baby in their fifth month to have at least one feeding during the night. Most parents at this age simply reduce the number of night feedings rather than eliminate them altogether.

## How to Gently Reduce Night Feeds

Since many babies do generally wake up in the night because they feel hungry and need to eat (especially in the first 6 months), it may be possible to shift some of their calorie intake to the daytime. This on its own can theoretically reduce night wakings and therefore improve night sleep.

If it does not, I recommend that you pick the feeding (or feedings) that you want to keep for the night—usually parents choose the one where the baby currently feeds the best. (You can use either a dream feed or a set time to keep this feeding—more on those shortly.) At this feeding, allow your baby to feed as much and long as they need. Once your baby is done eating, coach them back to sleep if needed.

You have two options for the other wakings:

- ✧ *Option 1* is to coach them back to sleep with no feeding for all of their wakings before 6 AM.
- ✧ *Option 2* is to feed your baby at their other wakings, but slowly (over the course of 3 to 4 nights) reduce the amount or duration of feeding until, eventually, you're not feeding them but rather coaching them back to sleep if they continue to wake. (If you are breastfeeding, gradually reduce the length of each feed, a few minutes at a time. If you are bottle feeding, gradually reduce the amount in the bottle by an ounce or more each night.) This is the more gradual approach. You'll remain cribside practicing the steps of the Modified Shuffle for each non-feeding waking.

  *Note*: If you try Option 2 and your baby starts to cry because they are "too awake" after their feeding, then you will be better off stopping this approach the next night and instead using Option 1 for all wakings aside from the one you wish to keep.

While you are reducing night feeds, be prepared to feed your baby more frequently during the day.

Some sleep experts suggest pushing a baby's feeding later and later each night in order to slowly lengthen their sleep stretches. I don't recommend this; I find that it leaves my parents exhausted, and this makes sleep coaching more difficult, because tired parents are less consistent. The only time I've seen this work is with night nannies or newborn care specialists who are in the home solely for the purpose of supporting the baby during the nighttime hours.

Now, let's talk about the one or two feedings that you plan to keep. There are two methods to try: dream feeds and set-time feeds.

### Dream Feeds

With a dream feed, you are feeding your baby before they wake and cry in an attempt to extend the length of the sleep stretch that follows. (For more on dream feeds, flip back to page 143.)

Bailey was 5½ months old when her parents contacted Gentle Sleep Coach Heather Irvine, CLEC, because they needed help with her night wakings. Before the 4-month sleep regression, she had slept 8 hours at the beginning of each night. During the regression, her parents went back to feeding her at night when she woke. When Heather started with this family, Bailey was waking three times a night to feed, and the parents wanted to get back to having that one longer stretch at night. "I had them establish some dream feed times," says Heather, "by going to Bailey 30 minutes before she usually woke in the middle of the night." Over the course of 10 days, Heather worked with Bailey's parents to reduce the first two feedings by 1 ounce every 2 nights. This strategy helped Bailey get back to her 8-hour stretch. It also helped her wean from two night feedings to only one. "Within 2 weeks the whole family was much more rested!" says Heather.

You can use dream feeds in conjunction with reducing ounces over the course of a few nights, like Heather suggested for Bailey's family. To do this, schedule one dream feed (offering the full amount of milk) and then reduce the ounces in the other feedings over the course of a few nights.

If you're considering multiple dream feeds, know that many parents have a difficult time setting an alarm past 1 AM for a second dream feed. We advise that if your baby wakes close to the next feeding time, just feed them and get them back to sleep as you normally would. If you keep two feedings at night, you can use a dream feed for around the time they first wake, and then feed them on the second waking only if it has been at least 3 hours since the dream feed.

### Set-Time Feeds

Some babies do not respond well to dream feeds and will not feed well, only to wake shortly afterward. If this sounds like your baby, we recommend using *set-time feeds*. With set-time feeds, you choose the time at which to feed your baby at night (around 10 PM for a first feeding, for instance, and around 2 AM for the second feeding, if you are keeping a second). For any other night wakings, you soothe your baby back to sleep without a feed.

If, for example, your baby wakes at 1 AM, you wouldn't let them cry until 2 AM and then feed them. Rather, you would coach them back to sleep and then feed them the next time they wake after 2 AM.

When the goal is to move from multiple feedings down to only one, I ask parents to look at their logs to see which night feeding is the one in which their baby takes in most of their nutrition. If they find that the 1 AM feed is the "biggest," I will suggest that their set-time feeding is the first waking after midnight. When their baby wakes anytime after midnight, they would feed them and put them back to bed, then coach them back to sleep without feeding for all other wakings.

It's okay if you need to reassure your baby back to sleep after a set time feeding. At the same time, it's okay if they fall asleep while feeding, too.

If you are breastfeeding, consider having another parent or caregiver coach your baby back to sleep at nonfeeding times, as it might be easier for your baby—they won't be expecting that person to nurse them.

### WHEN YOUR BABY NO LONGER NEEDS TO FEED AT NIGHT: WEANING ALL NIGHT FEEDINGS

If you have already weaned your baby off all feedings but one (and your pediatrician has confirmed that they are fine with none), to wean off their remaining feeding, I recommend a 4-night phaseout:

✩   Whether breastfeeding or bottle-feeding, feed your baby just once during the night for 3 nights, using either the set-time or dream feed option. Reduce the feeding amount at this last feeding over the course of these 3 nights (as Heather recommended to Bailey's parents on page 266). Don't feed them again until they wake around 6 AM. If they wake at other times, offer physical and verbal assurance to coach them back to sleep.

✩   On the fourth night, drop the feeding and comfort them back to sleep each time they wake. Use the guidelines for the Modified Shuffle (page 252) to soothe them, picking them up to calm them only if they get overly upset.

---

## Dramatic Wake-Up

When you start sleep coaching, you'll want to follow my "6 AM rule": any time your baby wakes before 6 AM, you'll coach them back to sleep as you would with any night waking. For example, if your baby wakes at 5:30 AM, you'll coach them back to sleep until 6 AM. If they are not asleep by 6 AM, then you can throw in the towel and do something I call *Dramatic Wake-Up*.

Dramatic Wake-Up simply helps your baby understand that nighttime is now over, and it is time to wake up for the day. Once you determine that your baby is not going to fall asleep again, do Dramatic Wake-Up:

- Stand up quickly.
- Leave the room.
- Count to ten.
- Enter the room again and perform the following routine:
  — Open the blinds.
  — Say "Good morning! Nighttime is over!" in an energetic voice.
  — Pick them up and leave the sleep area.

You don't want to simply pick up your baby to start the day because they will then assume that when they can't get back to sleep on their own, you'll just pick them up. Dramatic Wake-Up's separation time teaches your baby that they are instead being picked up because nighttime has ended.

*Note*: If your baby wakes early and you just can't make it until 6 AM, Dramatic Wake-Up is your next step then as well. And if you feel that, at 6 AM, your baby is close to falling back to sleep, feel free to coach them longer. Just make sure to wake them for the day around 7:30 AM to avoid throwing off your usual schedule.

## Weaning from the Pacifier during Sleep Coaching

Most pediatricians recommend weaning your child off the pacifier by 18 months to 2 years (I recommend starting even earlier—before 15 months), but if your baby is waking up a lot at night seeking their "paci," you might want to tackle it now. Be prepared for a few nights of unpleasantness as there is no gradual way to wean the pacifier. It's either in your baby's mouth or it's not.

As with most processes that I recommend, you'll want to start these steps at bedtime after a great day of naps. You'll put your baby down in their crib after their standard soothing pre-bed routine without their pacifier. Then follow the steps for the Modified Shuffle.

Knowing that your baby is missing the added comfort of their pacifier to soothe them back to sleep during nonfeeding night wakings, you may need to go a bit slower with the process.

As with Phase 1, your nap plan for Phase 2 is to fill your baby's daytime sleep tank any way you can.

## Phase 3: Nap Coaching

With nap coaching, the goal is the same as it is at bedtime: helping your baby learn how to fall asleep and put themselves back to sleep independently, but this time during daytime naps.

I usually work on nap coaching with babies after they are 6 months old, so don't be worried if your baby isn't yet ready to learn how to put themselves to sleep on their own for naps. If your baby is now a pro at going to sleep and back to sleep by themselves at night, however, you may be ready to apply the Modified Shuffle to daytime naps.

You also might choose to nap coach if your baby's sleep crutch is no longer working—even if you are still not "done" coaching them at night. If your baby is not sleeping well during the day, nighttime coaching might be even more of a challenge.

If you do plan to nighttime and nap coach concurrently, always coach first at bedtime (and then throughout the night) and do your first nap coaching the following morning. Babies learn best at bedtime after a day of successful naps.

But be forewarned that concurrent nighttime and nap coaching may not work for alert babies because it is a lot of change all at once. At a minimum, you may have to look at how fast you go with these little ones. You might have to just focus on nights while you do anything you can to get them their daytime sleep.

Before we start, I'd like to acknowledge that embarking on sleep coaching at nap time can seem a bit daunting. When families are at the stage where they are getting naps "any way you can get 'em," they sometimes have more schedule flexibility—they might be able to head out for an afternoon at the park where baby sleeps comfortably in the stroller. When you start nap coaching, you need to commit to being at home for the process. It can also sometimes feel like the coaching process is all that you're doing all day. But I assure you that the time spent is worth it!

SLEEP COACHING AT NAP TIME

The nap coaching process is fairly similar to bedtime and middle-of-the-night coaching. You'll start by putting your baby down in their sleep space "calm but awake" and then follow the same steps you used when you coached them at bedtime. However, here are a few key suggestions that apply specifically to naps:

- ✭ Start sleep coaching at the onset of the first nap of the day. Your baby will have an easier time falling asleep in the morning than later on.

- ✭ At this age, your baby is probably taking three or four naps per day. Try to get your baby down for a nap in their crib for at least two of these naps. I find that coaching at more than two naps a day can feel a bit overwhelming, so if you need to nap your baby in a stroller or a carrier for the remaining nap(s), that's just fine—particularly if you get to 2 or 3 PM and your logs show that your baby is short on sleep. You'll want to make sure you've filled your baby's daytime sleep tank so that they are not overtired at bedtime.

- ✭ Make sure to follow your usual pre-nap-time routine first, so your baby knows that a nap is coming next.

- ✭ Start by coaching next to your baby's crib.

- ✭ Follow the same steps you used when using the Modified Shuffle at bedtime. With nap coaching, however, you'll move farther away every 3 days, even if your baby didn't nap well on that day.

- ✭ Ideally try to spend around an hour coaching your baby to sleep, if needed (and use Dramatic Wake-Up if you get to the end of the hour and they are not asleep; see box on page 268). If an hour feels impossible, try for 30 minutes. Stay by your baby's crib and follow the guidelines for the Modified Shuffle.

- ✭ If your baby wakes before the 45-minute mark, or seems tired and cranky when they awake, try to coach your baby back to sleep. If they haven't fallen back asleep after 15 to 30 minutes, you can move on to Dramatic Wake-Up.

Your nap coaching will have four possible outcomes:

1.  Your baby responds well to nap coaching, goes to sleep within the hour, and naps for more than 45 minutes. Yay!

2.  Your baby takes only a 45-minute nap but wakes rested. (Be sure to watch their sleepy cues and the clock after this, because they may be ready for their next nap early.)

3.  Your baby sleeps for less than 45 minutes. I call these abbreviated naps "disaster naps." Your baby has not gone through a complete sleep cycle and will often wake cranky and tired. (As with a 45-minute nap, be sure to watch their sleepy cues and the clock after this, because they may be ready for their next nap early.)

4.  Your baby doesn't go to sleep at all, despite your coaching. Leave the room and perform Dramatic Wake-Up. After no sleep, their next nap will come sooner, so keep your eye out for sleepy cues.

---

## Dramatic Wake-Up at Nap Time

When you first try nap coaching, you may find that you have been trying to get your baby to sleep for over 30 minutes and have a gut feeling that they just won't be going to sleep! You may get the same feeling when trying to coach them *back* to sleep from a mid-nap wake-up; after 15 to 30 minutes with no success, they are unlikely to fall asleep again. In both cases, rather than continuing to try to get them to sleep, I suggest ending the nap with Dramatic Wake-Up, the same way you would if your baby won't fall back to sleep in the morning before their standard wake time.

Dramatic Wake-Up tells your baby that nap time is now over. You don't want to simply stop coaching and pick them up because they will then associate enough protest over going back to sleep with being picked up. Instead, follow the directions that you learned on page 268: When you enter the room, open the blinds to let the sunshine in and say, "Nap time is over!" in an energetic voice.

Sometimes I suggest that parents first focus on coaching for just the morning nap and add coaching for the second nap only once they feel they are making progress during the morning nap. I recommend this for my parents who feel overwhelmed when they think about coaching for more than one nap and also those who worry they can't be consistent. Plus, successfully coaching during the morning nap can give you the much-needed win you need to feel confident moving on to the next nap.

For more on nap coaching, please see my book *The Sleep Lady's Good Night, Sleep Tight.*

## Co-Sleeping in Month 5

Is co-sleeping working for you at night? I always say that if it's not broken, don't try to fix it! It's important to know, however, that even though you're co-sleeping you can still sleep coach, and still benefit from doing so. We'll address how to use the Modified Shuffle whether you are bedsharing or room sharing, as well as how to move your little one out of the family bed if you feel that it is time.

### Co-Sleeping and Sleep Coaching

Many parents are happily co-sleeping with their babies but would like to sleep coach to improve everyone's sleep. Sleep coaching can be especially helpful at bedtime, so that you don't have to go to bed at 7 PM!

The approach below assumes that your baby sleeps in a co-sleeper attached to your bed, because that is the style of co-sleeping that my team and I recommend—particularly if you will be leaving your sleeping baby unattended until you come to bed. If you are bedsharing and want to improve your baby's bedtime, but not go to bed at the same time as your baby, you'll need to come up with a safe plan for where your baby will sleep when you're out of the room. (Keep reading for how to modify this process if you are room sharing with your baby in a crib.)

Here is how to adapt the first steps of the Modified Shuffle for your little co-sleeper:

1. Go through your usual bedtime routine in your room.

2. If you normally nurse your baby to sleep, start nursing—sitting upright in your bed **with the light on**. Gently unlatch your baby when they are done feeding, and burp them.

3. Put your baby in their co-sleeper, with the railing up, "calm but awake."

4. Dim the lights.

5. Lie down next to the co-sleeper and intermittently pat and shush your baby to sleep. Remember, it's okay to pick up your baby to calm them—see page 255 for the Modified Shuffle guidelines.

---

## Sleep Coaching Baby Steps for Co-Sleeping

If moving straight from nursing your baby to sleep to just patting them intermittently feels too fast, you can slow this process down a step by starting with not allowing them to suck to sleep. Instead, lay your baby next to you and pat, shush, and snuggle or spoon them to sleep. The next night you can do the same, but move a bit farther away while still patting and shushing. Once your baby is asleep, put them in their co-sleeper and raise the railing. Eventually, you'll get to the point where you can put your baby directly into the co-sleeper after feeding them to begin the Modified Shuffle.

---

Once you have mastered putting your baby into the co-sleeper and patting and shushing them only intermittently to sleep, you can continue sleep coaching by following the step-by-step Modified Shuffle, with a few minor adjustments:

1. At bedtime, put your baby down in the co-sleeper "calm but awake."

2. Start by sitting next to the co-sleeper (with the railings up), either on the bed or in a chair on the other side of the co-sleeper.

3. Follow the Modified Shuffle guidelines. Return to the bed or chair to soothe your baby each time they wake but doing less and less each night—at bedtime and again each time your baby wakes *before* you want to go to bed yourself. Do this for 3 nights.

4. Then, on night 4, move the chair away from the co-sleeper halfway to the door or at the door (depending on the room setup), and use only your voice to soothe them. (This step will be very difficult to do if you were using a lot of touch during the first 3 nights.)

5. For wakings that occur *before* your bedtime, coach your baby back to sleep from your chair position.

6. For wakings that occur *after* your bedtime (and *after* the time you set for a dream feed or between set time feedings, if that is part of your plan), coach your baby back to sleep from your bed, patting and shushing them to sleep, with a focus on doing less patting and shushing over time. You can also do a cribside check if necessary.

If your baby co-sleeps in your bed, you may choose to start them in a co-sleeper and then bring them into bed with you for the rest of the night. If your plan is to move them to their own room eventually, you may wish to keep them in their co-sleeper.

If you are room sharing with your baby in a crib, simply follow the standard steps of the Modified Shuffle where you start by standing by the crib and continue on to the chair. Once you've moved away from the crib, you can still do a cribside check when they wake, but then do your remaining verbal reassurance from your bed.

An alternative option is to start with the crib right next to your bed (like a co-sleeper) and every few nights move the crib farther away from the bed. You can either use the bed as the "chair" in the Modified Shuffle or introduce a chair in order to move even farther away from the crib for the last few nights of the Modified Shuffle. Again, the final step will be giving any additional verbal reassurance from your bed.

As long as you've taken your baby's safety into account, you can adjust the Modified Shuffle in any way that works for you.

## Moving Out of the Family Bed

You may have looked at co-sleeping this month and decided that it is no longer working for you. Or you may be dealing with "reactive co-sleeping," where your baby ends up in your bed out of desperation because you are simply trying to get more sleep for you both. Co-sleeping may not be a choice or a philosophical commitment for you—it may just feel like the only way you can get your baby to sleep at bedtime or back to sleep when they wake at night.

If you've decided it's time to move your baby to their own sleep space permanently, I recommend the following process:

### Stage 1: Daytime and Playtime

If you haven't done so already, have your baby spend time in their room during the day—playing, being read to, getting changed. Make the experience positive. You can also feed them in their room before taking them to yours at bedtime, to further acclimate them to the space.

### Stage 2: Nap Time

If your baby is not yet napping in their own room, have them start. You can start by napping with them for a few days on a mattress you bring in for a short time. Even just co-sleeping with them in their room is progress. You can then use the Super Slow Shuffle process to help them fall asleep in their crib. If this feels too abrupt, just put them to sleep as you normally would for naps and skip to Stage 3 to focus on night sleep first.

### Stage 3: Nighttime

In this stage, you start by co-sleeping with your baby on a mattress in your baby's room for a few nights to create a bridge from the family bed to the crib. Then you follow the steps of the Modified Shuffle with your baby in the crib just as you would have had you not been co-sleeping. You can start at bedtime only or you can coach them back to sleep after all wakings.

Some parents choose to night wean (whether entirely, or from two or three nightly feedings down to one) while they are co-sleeping on the mattress in their baby's room, before beginning the Modified Shuffle. If you have been breastfeeding at night, it can be helpful to have the non-breastfeeding parent be the one to co-sleep with the baby and have the feeding parent only come in to nurse for the wakings that require feeding.

If you are trying to move away from "reactive co-sleeping," it is particularly important to stay consistent while following the Modified Shuffle. Having your little one stay in their crib when they wake at 2 AM, 3 AM, and 4 AM but bringing them into your bed at 5 AM sends them mixed messages and may encourage them to cry or fuss longer in the future. I suggest coaching them back to sleep in the crib each time they wake up until 6 AM. Then you can use Dramatic Wake-Up if you don't think they'll get back to sleep before their usual morning wake time.

## Continuing to Co-Sleep

If co-sleeping is working well for your family, I recommend remaining in Phase 1 of Baby-Led Sleep Coaching, rather than moving on to Phase 2. You can sleep coach at bedtime by putting your baby in a crib or co-sleeper, but then, after your little one's first wake-up, you can bring them into your bed for the rest of the night. This will allow you to put your baby to sleep at their bedtime without having to go to bed yourself.

## Moving on to Nap Coaching

If your baby is able to put themselves to sleep in the co-sleeper at bedtime and also back to sleep throughout the night, it may be time to start nap coaching. You can follow the Modified Shuffle steps for your little co-sleepers at nap time as well.

You may choose to nap coach your baby in their own sleep space to allow them to safely nap throughout the day without you, before sleep coaching at night. I find, however, that nap coaching when a baby has not first been coached back to sleep at night can be a bit more difficult.

## Create Your Sleep Coaching Plan

Now it's time to design your sleep-coaching plan! I always encourage parents to create their plan during the waking hours. Think it through, talk it through, and write it down. Putting your plan on paper will ensure that you're both on the same page (literally and figuratively!) and help you avoid miscommunication. Most important, it will help you be consistent with your child.

I have developed a PDF template you can use to create your plan. It's available on my website at SleepLady.com/SleepPlan.

Before you begin, make sure that you can set aside 3 weeks to commit to your sleep coaching plan. You'll want enough time to ensure that you can get through the suggested number of nights for each step of the Modified Shuffle. You'll also want some extra time in case you decide to spend a few extra days at one or two of the steps.

Consider, too, what's going on in your lives. Has one of you just returned to work? Is there any extra stress you're dealing with? Life changes or additional stress can impact your ability to be consistent in following your plan.

You also want to ensure that you and your partner are in agreement, and that you trust your ability to present a united front as you sleep coach. Confirm that everyone involved in the plan is on board and that you have the support you need.

The following is a sample plan, using the template, for 5-month-old Marion, who sleeps in a crib.

# Our Sleep Plan for: Marion

We met with our pediatrician and discussed our baby's eating, growth, and general health. We have ruled out any potential underlying medical conditions that may be interfering with Marion's sleep. Our pediatrician has given us the green light to begin sleep coaching.

After reviewing her sleep averages, we have found that our baby requires on average the following amount of sleep:

| | |
|---|---|
| **Total amount of nighttime sleep:** | 11 hours |
| **Total amount of daytime sleep:** | 3.5–4 hours |
| **Number of naps:** | 3, sometimes 4 |

After reviewing my baby's eating and sleep logs over the last few days, we believe their natural bedtime window is: around 7 PM

We will be working toward an approximate eating and sleeping schedule as outlined below:

| | |
|---|---|
| 6 AM–7:30 AM | Wake-up range |
| | Feeding |
| 8:30 AM–9 AM | Nap (8 am at the earliest) |
| | Feeding |
| Around 12 or 1 PM | Nap |
| | Feeding |
| Around 3 or 4 PM | Nap |
| | Feeding |
| | *Possible fourth nap if her daytime sleep tank hasn't been filled |
| 6 PM–6:30 PM | Start bedtime routine |
| | Feeding |
| 7 PM | Start the first step of the Modified Shuffle |
| | Feeding |

## OUR BEDTIME ROUTINE WILL INCLUDE THE FOLLOWING:

1. Bath (every few nights) or gentle sponge bath.
2. Massage.
3. Nurse with the night-light on.
4. Short song or book.
5. Into crib awake.

## OUR BEDTIME PLAN:

- Dad will sit by the crib until Marion falls asleep.
- Dad has reviewed all the rules of the Modified Shuffle.
- Dad will decide when it is appropriate to pick up Marion to calm her and will determine if it helps her.
- Mom will not coach Dad from the doorway and will support his efforts, knowing that he loves Marion and is a caring father to her.
- Mom and Dad agree that learning to put yourself to sleep is an essential life skill and that it is one of our tasks as parents to teach Marion.

## OUR POSITIONS WILL BE AS FOLLOWS:

- Nights 1–3: Standing by the crib.
- Nights 4–6: Sitting on a chair 2 feet from the crib.
- Nights 7–9: Sitting on a chair 3-plus feet from the crib (moving 1 foot farther away each night).

## OUR NIGHTTIME STRATEGY:

- We and the pediatrician agree that Marion needs one feeding during an 11–12-hour night.
- We will feed her at the first waking after midnight and then not until 6 AM at the earliest, and then we will start our day.

- For her first feeding, Mom will go in, change Marion's diaper, nurse her, and place her back in the crib. (Mom will unlatch her once she is done with her feeding and not allow her to suckle back to sleep.)
- For her second feeding, Mom will go in, change Marion's diaper, and nurse her for incrementally less time over the course of 3 nights (until the fourth night, when she will be coached back to sleep with no second feeding).
- Dad will go in and sit next to Marion's crib at each waking before and after each feeding, and follow the Modified Shuffle steps.
- We will not bring Marion out of her room to start the day before 6 AM.
- We will not bring Marion back into our bed.

## OUR NAP PLAN:

We have decided not to nap coach at this time.

- We will fill Marion's daytime sleep tank by getting her naps any way we can.
- We will rock her to sleep and put her to sleep in her crib.
- If she doesn't fall asleep easily, we will put her in the front carrier and let her sleep there for her nap.

## OUR DAYCARE PROVIDER HAS AGREED TO THE FOLLOWING:

She will make sure that Marion gets 4 hours of daytime naps even if she has to sleep in the stroller or in someone's arms. We shared with her Marion's schedule and average wakeful window length (1½ hours), and she is willing to work with us on the timing of her day naps.

We're ready to go! We have blocked out 3 weeks of our schedule and are dedicating ourselves to improving our baby's sleep habits! There is sleep for all at the end of the tunnel!

As you fill out your sleep coaching plan, here are a few things to keep in mind:

☆   Focus on nights first. Daytime sleep is harder and develops later, so don't fret if your baby still needs help sleeping for naps (or is even still napping in the swing!).

☆   Even though you're focusing on nights first, have a plan for daytime sleep. At this age, it's important to help your baby get daytime sleep any way you can. Where will your baby nap and how will you get them to sleep?

☆   Review your feeding log with your doctor and ask about your baby's nighttime feeding needs. How many will you include in your plan?

☆   Decide how you will address night wakings and night feedings. How many feedings did you and your pediatrician decide your baby needs at night? How will you address night wakings that are not tied to feedings? Will you be focusing on bedtime only, or night wakings as well?

☆   Take your baby's temperament into account. How will this affect your plan?

---

## Consistency Is Key

Remember, babies (and adults) thrive on consistency. Once you're ready to start following your sleep plan, make sure you're able to stick with it. Sleep coaching takes time, patience, and parental perseverance.

---

## Sleep Coaching Challenges

Often the solution to sleep coaching challenges is to slow the process down a bit, staying with one or more steps for an extra day or two. For other challenges, we have specific suggestions.

### Need to Take a Break?

If, after 30 minutes (or even just 15) of the Modified Shuffle method, you're feeling like you can't take your baby's crying or the stress of the process, you should stop. You want to be in a place where you can commit to following through. If your heart is telling you to stop, you won't be able to be consistent.

And that's okay! You can take a break. And that break can be as long or as short as you need. You could try the next day. Or you could give yourself some time to think about it, and wait to start again once you are feeling like you can commit.

If you feel that the Modified Shuffle is too much but want to move beyond sleep shaping, you could try the Super Slow Shuffle outlined in Month 4. Or, you can try the Jiggle and Soothe (or Jiggle and Soothe 2.0) so that you feel you're making some progress without doing full-on sleep coaching by following the Modified Shuffle.

> If you've followed your plan for 3 to 5 nights without seeing any improvement, you should stop. It is possible that your baby is not ready for sleep coaching (or might even have an underlying medical condition that is making the process too difficult). Assess the situation before deciding when to start trying again.

## Overstimulation While Sleep Coaching

I've had parents tell me that they feel that their baby is getting "overstimulated" by the parents' presence next to them as they are being coached to sleep. While this *can* happen, I find that it is rare. Parents are often experiencing this additional crying as they sleep coach their baby and are trying to interpret what it means. Sometimes it can be crying from frustration: "I don't understand why you are no longer rocking me to sleep!" "I don't know how to do this. Why don't you pick me up and feed me to sleep?" But yes, sometimes, in an effort to soothe their babies, the parents unintentionally do "too much," and move too quickly from one soothing tool to the next, and this makes their baby more upset. I recommend slowing down and using the SOAR process to see which soothing tools are truly working.

## Early Rising

Have you started sleep coaching and your baby is now taking a much longer stretch at the beginning of the night, but is now waking, still tired, at 4 or 5 AM? Early rising is a very common sleep struggle!

Early rising is not the same as having an *early bird*—a little one who wakes refreshed but earlier than their parents would like. Early risers are not happy when they wake at the crack of dawn. They are awake but grouchy because their nighttime sleep tank was not sufficiently filled.

There are five main causes of early rising:

1. Your baby experienced too long of a wakeful window between their last nap of the day and bedtime.
2. Your baby's nap tank was not filled the day before.
3. Your baby went to bed too late.
4. Your baby was put down too drowsy at bedtime.
5. Your baby is hungry and not quite ready to go all night without a feeding.

You'll notice that the first three causes all contribute to overtiredness. As you'll recall, when a baby is overtired at bedtime, they'll often—counter to what might seem logical—wake earlier than usual. As you'll also remember, bedtime is the easiest time for your baby to learn to put themselves to sleep independently. If they are put to sleep too drowsy, they are not given the opportunity to master this skill, and it will be even harder for them to get themselves back to sleep at 5 AM.

## How to Help Early Risers

In order to help nip early rising in the bud, you'll want to treat early wake-ups like any other night waking and coach your baby back to sleep. If they do not fall back to sleep by 6 AM, go ahead and do Dramatic Wake-Up.

Whether they get back to sleep or not, your job that day will be to fill your baby's daytime sleep tank, to try to keep early rising from occurring again the next morning. You'll want to make sure that your baby doesn't nap before 8 AM, so that you don't reinforce early rising by throwing off your schedule for the day. You'll also want to watch your baby's sleepy cues and pay attention to the length of the last wakeful window of the day to make sure that it's not too long, so that they are not too overtired by bedtime.

If the early rising persists, be sure to commit to coaching your baby back to sleep. Early rising will improve with persistence and consistency. Hang in there!

## Daycare and Sleep Coaching

I don't recommend that you start sleep coaching when your baby is about to start attending daycare. It is too much change at once! Wait until your baby has settled in to daycare (there is no set time, but many parents feel it takes 3 to 6 weeks) and you feel that with their particular temperament, sleep coaching won't be too much for them.

Even with a baby who has been in daycare for a bit, sleep coaching can be challenging. Some parents find that their babies don't nap well when they are there (and so their daytime sleep tank is not filled). Some daycares don't have a nap schedule, or a baby has difficulty sleeping in the daycare environment. I've also had parents tell me that their daycare claims their baby is not tired enough for a nap. But as you've learned, when babies don't sleep well during the day, they often don't sleep well at night. And some babies refuse a bottle during the day, leading to reverse cycling and waking up more often to feed at night, to take in the extra calories that they missed.

As you know, I always tell parents to start sleep coaching after a fantastic day of naps so that their baby is happy and not overtired at bedtime. If your baby hasn't been sleeping well at daycare, you may, for instance, want to start sleep coaching on a Saturday night after a day of holding your baby for naps. You can then follow your plan, seeing if starting with 2 weekend days of solid napping helps jump-start the process.

We also suggest that you work with the daycare to solve napping issues. You can:

- ✵ Share your sleep coaching plan with them and see if they will work with you and your baby's needs. Share the schedule you find your baby does best on. When you drop your baby off each day, tell the daycare what time your baby woke and when you think they will need their next nap.
- ✵ Ask them if they can follow a suggested schedule (within reason).
- ✵ Have them fill your baby's daytime sleep tank any way they—safely— can (that is, not simply allowing them to nap unattended in a swing).

The goal is a baby that is relatively well rested at pick up, ready to face bedtime and the night ahead. Please see our Daycare suggestions in the Appendix.

## If You Have a One-Bedroom Apartment

Some families room share with their babies not because they want to but because the size or layout of their home doesn't offer any alternative. The good news is that you can still sleep coach.

You can start with the crib either next to your bed or several feet away. If it's next to your bed, over the course of three nights, move the crib progressively farther away. If the crib is already away from the bed, start by placing a chair next to it.

At this point, follow the standard steps of the Modified Shuffle, where you start by standing or sitting by the crib. Once you've moved away from the crib, you can still do a brief cribside check when they wake, but then do your remaining verbal reassurance from your bed.

If your baby is very sensitive to your presence in the room, you can also try the following to minimize disruption:

- ✮  A screen divider placed between their crib and your bed.
- ✮  White noise to block out the sounds of you moving around the room while they are asleep.
- ✮  A SlumberPod, a tentlike contraption that creates total darkness and a sense of a separate space for your baby to sleep in.

If you need to get up in the morning before your baby wakes, we recommend leaving out your clothes and other necessary items in another room, so that your getting ready does not disturb your baby's sleep.

---

### Sharing a Room with a Sibling

If possible, I wouldn't recommend putting your baby in with a sibling until they are sleeping through the night. It's not worth the risk of your baby waking their sibling at this stage and adding another family member to the list of those not sleeping.

 Feeling overwhelmed? One of our Gentle Sleep Coaches would love to help you create your sleep plan and support you as you coach your baby through it! Visit FindaSleepCoach.com.

## YOUR SELF-CARE

While you're teaching your child self-regulation through sleep coaching, it helps if you are also self-regulated. As we learned in Start Here, because of the power of mirror neurons, being calm and self-regulated helps our babies self-regulate.[117]

It's even more important at this time to make sure that you are getting enough sleep, and that you're caring for your body with light exercise and movement and your mind with meditation.

Ziva Meditation expert Emily Fletcher says that when her life is particularly full, she is even more disciplined about her meditation. "Meditation isn't a cute thing that you do when you have extra time . . . because *no one* has extra time," she says. "It's the thing that you do to optimize your brain, which is what imprints every cell in your body and makes every single decision in your life. If you're not taking the time to optimize this machine, what else are you doing with your time?"

Flip back through the previous five chapters and pick one or two self-care practices that you can commit to today. Then make a self-care plan for yourself that goes along with your sleep coaching plan.

Remember, at the end of the day, you are in control of the decisions regarding your baby's sleep, and how you help them grow. I think that most "parental guilt" occurs when well-meaning family or friends offer advice (or even judgment) about your sleep coaching choices.

It can be difficult to hear your mom, best friend, sister, or neighbor question, correct, or give unsolicited advice about how you are caring for your child (especially if both you and baby are short on sleep and patience). During these times, it's important to remember that **you are an amazing, caring parent**. You've made the choices you have for a reason.

If you find that your loved ones are questioning your choice to sleep coach (especially if they are proponents of "cry it out"), don't feel the need to explain yourself. If you must explain why you are choosing to sleep coach, give your family member a copy of this book or direct them to my blog (SleepLady.com). That way they can digest the information from a source other than you—which, for them, might lend your chosen approach more credibility.

Don't forget to remind yourself that you know your baby best. If your baby is cranky and rubbing their eyes, you know that they need sleep, and soon. Even if your dad is urging you to let them stay up "just a little bit longer," you know that it's best to go with your instincts and the lessons that you've learned while sleep coaching. Rather than ignore your instincts because of other parties' advice, **trust your gut**.

If all else fails, blame it on The Sleep Lady! I've got your back.

## ONE-PAGE FAST TO SLEEP SUMMARY

**Month 5 Theme:** *Are you and your baby ready for gentle sleep coaching? Here's how to get started.*

### What to Focus on This Month

1. Soothe your baby's stranger anxiety with our tips on page 238.
2. Feed your newly distractible eater in a quiet room to help them avoid snacking and not eating enough during the day, which can lead to increased feedings at night.
3. If you feel like you are still recovering from the 4-month sleep regression, revisit our Baby-Led Sleep Shaping elements on page 218 to get back on track.
4. Is your baby ready to start Baby-Led Sleep Coaching?
   - Revisit the Sleep-Coaching Readiness Checklist on page 222.
   - Get the green light from your pediatrician to start sleep coaching and review your baby's eating if you plan to wean night feedings.
   - Create your sleep plan, including how you will address night feedings.
   - Decide how you will fill your baby's daytime sleep tank— including if your baby is in daycare.
   - Make sure you have set aside 3 weeks to focus on this process— ideally without any traveling with your baby.
5. Make a "self-care plan" for yourself that goes along with your sleep coaching plan. Pick one or two self-care practices that you can commit to today.

### What Not to Worry About

Forty-five-minute naps, plus nap coaching and weaning all-night feeds if it feels like too much to take on at once (and particularly if a parent has recently started back to work).

---

For a printable PDF of this month's FAST to Sleep Summary plus helpful book bonuses, go to SleepLady.com/NewbornSleepGuide.

# What's Next?

*The Sleep Lady shares what you can look forward to in the coming months.*

Congratulations! You've made it through the newborn months! Be proud of what you and your baby have accomplished so far. You've come a long way!

Each month you've learned what you can realistically expect from your baby. You'll continue to keep tabs on what your baby is capable of as they grow. For the next several months, you may have to let family members know that your baby naps best at home (which supports better sleep at night). After gentle sleep coaching, I find that parents and caregivers become very protective of their baby's sleep and schedule and will guard it like the gold that it is!

You may be excited about the sleep progress you've made over the last several months. Or you may feel disappointed because you had hoped to be further along. We get it! Sometimes things don't go as planned because babies arrive prematurely, experience feeding challenges, develop medical conditions, reach milestones at later times, or have more intense temperaments. There are a lot of variabilities when it comes to babies under 6 months! If you need additional support, consider hiring one of our Gentle Sleep Coaches for one-on-one sleep support. You can set up a consult at FindaSleepCoach.com.

Things will change quite a bit for the better regarding sleep in the next 6 months. Your baby's sleep patterns will be even more regular—particularly with your gentle guidance. If sleep challenges do come up, or if you're just looking for gentle sleep coaching techniques appropriate for older babies, I've got a lot of suggestions for you in *The Sleep Lady's Good Night, Sleep Tight.*

Learning how to fall asleep independently can be hard even with a gentle, responsive approach! I remind parents that while it's their job to help their baby stay regulated, it isn't their responsibility to keep their baby from experiencing frustration altogether. It's natural for a child to get frustrated during sleep coaching. When we go through the process with them, we help them move through the discomfort of letting go of external soothing (like being held and rocked to sleep) and learning to rely on their own skills.

Remembering that frustration isn't the same as dysregulation can help you sit with your baby's crying even as you are trying to soothe them. Manageable frustration is the foundation of learning and actually helps babies rather than hinders them. It is the foundation of learning for you as a parent, as well. The trick is not to avoid frustration, but to support your baby through reassurance while they learn how to handle it.

Your baby learns best when they can feel the frustration but also have you nearby to support them as they learn to move through it. It is a dance that you two will do for years to come, especially as your child grows older and you encounter new parenting challenges. Your ability to participate in this dance requires self-reflection, patience, and a willingness to let go and let your child struggle and grow. Our children are often our best teachers, if we allow them to be.

Thank you for the honor of accompanying you on your parenting journey as we experienced these first 5 precious months together. My wish is for you to feel empowered as your baby's expert while making yourself a priority as well.

During this time in your baby's life you might feel like you are going it solo, but I assure you that you are not alone! My Gentle Sleep Coach Team and I are here for you!

Sweet dreams,
Kim

# Appendix

## PLANNING TO RETURN TO WORK

Going back to work can be challenging. There is a lot to manage! Any change in the family schedule can disrupt sleep, and having one or both parents heading back to work is a major change. My Gentle Sleep Coaches and I have found that families with a plan experience less sleep disruption. A plan can also help you keep your baby's sleep shaping foundation solid, so that you are ready for sleep coaching when the time is right.

### If You're Breastfeeding

Gentle Sleep Coach Heather Irvine, CLEC, finds that nursing mothers who make a plan for how to return to work and know ahead of time how they will manage to continue breastfeeding have a smoother transition.

To prepare your baby for their own transition, Gentle Sleep Coach Brandi Jordan, MSW, IBCLC, recommends introducing a bottle at no later than 6 weeks old (but after breastfeeding has been fully established). Waiting longer tends to cause confusion and make it harder for your baby to adjust.

## Suggestions for before Transitioning Back to Work

1. Address any lingering medical issues or questions so that you are not trying to handle those while also transitioning your baby to a new routine. For example, make sure that your baby's reflux is being addressed and they are feeding well.

2. Resolve any lingering day-night confusion. (See page 100 for tips.)

3. Start waking your baby at the appropriate time 2 weeks before you actually go back to work, to get them acclimated to the new schedule.

4. Schedule a "practice week" before you return to work to determine if you need to make any adjustments. For example, wake up at the time you'll need to wake for work and get showered and ready. Have the baby's bag packed and ready to go, and head out the door for a morning errand. You can also practice by starting daycare part-time.

5. If you intend to pump, have a plan—ideally, prepare to pump every 3 to 4 hours at work around the same times your baby would normally eat.

6. Arrange for some extra bonding time with your baby in the evenings and when you are off work.

Also, prepare yourself for potential sleep disruptions due to the change in routines. It is common for babies to initiate more night feedings at first, as they are looking for additional chances to bond and also may not be eating as well at daycare or with a new caregiver. (If you find that your baby is reverse cycling—feeding more at night than during the day—check out page 166.)

## Tips for Creating a Transition Plan

☆ If you are planning to pump (or, if you work from home, take breaks to nurse), have a meeting with your Human Resources department. Ask them for information on the company's policies regarding issues related to a breastfeeding employee's return to work. It is also helpful for you to review your rights according to your state. The Federal Patient Protection and Affordable Care Act of 2010, section 4207, states that any employer with fifty or more employees must provide nursing mothers with "reasonable break time" and a private space that is not a bathroom to pump milk until the employee's child turns 12 months old. Employers with fewer than fifty employees must also comply with the law unless they can provide reasonable proof that doing so would cause the company undue hardship or expense.

☆ Ask about flexible work schedules, part-time opportunities, or work-at-home options (allowing you to transition back to work gradually, creating less disruption in your family's schedule). If you plan on returning to work full-time, ask if you can return on Thursday or Friday that first week. Find out if you can work shorter weeks the first few weeks back, or take Wednesdays off. This can be a great way for you and your baby to adjust and give you ample time to reconnect every few days.

☆ Make sure to begin making caregiving arrangements before you go back to work. If you are going to be hiring a nanny, have them start at least a week or two before you return to work. This can help everyone adjust to the new schedule and establish a nice routine before you add work responsibilities to the mix. If you decide to use a daycare center, ask if you can bring your baby on a part-time basis for a week or two before you go back to work. This will give your baby time to get used to their new environment and caregiver.

# QUESTIONS TO ASK HOME-BASED NANNIES OR PROFESSIONAL DAYCARES

When you're working on a strong sleep shaping foundation, and especially if you've moved on to sleep coaching, quality naps are a big part of helping the process succeed. And if your baby is with a nanny or at a daycare during the day, someone else will be responsible for filling your baby's daytime sleep tank. You will want to review your sleep routines and share your baby's sleep cues, so they can support the healthy sleep habits you have started to put into place.

Before hiring an in-home caregiver or committing to a daycare, you'll want to find out how they approach daytime sleep. When evaluating daycare options, make sure to also take their sleep environment into account, as your newborn will be spending a lot of time napping during the day.

### Questions for Daycare Providers and Nannies

- ✡  What do you do regarding sleep?
- ✡  What if my baby cries?
- ✡  What are your rules on crying and sleeping?

### Questions for Daycare Providers Only

- ✡  Where and in what will my baby sleep?
- ✡  Is the nap area sleep-inducing? Is it a space separate from the noise and activity of non-nappers/older children? Are there room-darkening shades?
- ✡  What is your nap schedule?

# Acknowledgments

Words cannot express how grateful I am to my writer, Berit, who listened to me for hours on end about my passions, struggles, and wishes for parents of young babies. As a gentle parenting advocate herself who spent years co-sleeping with her little ones (one of whom was and still is alert), she understood me and helped pull out my gentle message for this young age group. As you probably know by now, I am not a big supporter of one-size-fits-all approaches (and especially not for newborns), and Berit was patient, caring, compassionate, and helped me crystalize my vision and message. She helped me birth the Baby-Led Sleep Shaping and Coaching approach you learned about in this book. Berit has been my ever-loving, supportive, and empowering "book midwife."

A special thank-you to Sam Horn for helping me focus my book proposal and introducing me to Berit. And an additional thanks to Berit's husband, Joey Coleman (accomplished author of *Never Lose a Customer Again*), who introduced me to Jim Levine, my literary agent, who has been my supporter from the beginning. I look forward to working on future books with Jim. His wise, kind, and gentle energy calms me and always makes me feel supported.

I could not have picked a better publisher for this book than BenBella Books. They are open-minded, creative, and empower me as an author! It has been so easy to work with them. Our editor Leah is detail-oriented, open-minded, and as a mother herself is thinking about her own experience! It's a lot of work to write a book, but with the BenBella team it flowed easily.

Thank you to Zvezdo, my children, and friends who have lovingly asked me about this book and who have given up time with me so I could spend that time writing. Thank you for your support and patience and for always believing in me.

I have been so honored throughout the past 25-plus years of helping parents with their children's sleep to meet amazing experts in related fields—from pediatricians to psychologists in PMADs to sleep medicine doctors to occupational therapists . . . the list goes on. Over the years I have had the privilege of referring back to these colleagues and sometimes just calling and chatting to problem-solve on how we can better serve parents, then later venturing into discussions about our own lives, deepening our connections.

Twelve years ago I started training people to be Gentle Sleep Coaches and help families all over the world by offering parents a gentle approach to sleep. Many of these coaches have contributed to this book and shared their own expertise as lactation consultants, night doulas, pediatricians, and researchers. I continue to learn from them each day and am so grateful that they have joined me on my mission.

These connections and friendships have been one of my deepest blessings and a great honor in my career and personal life. These bright lights of my village have reminded me that I am always learning, that we can be a village of support to each other, that we all struggle at times in parenting, and that, if we let ourselves, we can allow others to pick us up and support us in the joyous yet challenging journey of parenting.

At times or perhaps often it can seem that this parenting world is divided and filled with judgment—I hear and see this. Listening to all these amazing members of my Gentle Sleep Village, I am reminded that we are more united than we are divided.

We love our children and want the best for them. And we are searching for options and approaches that align with our values and parenting philosophies.

Although we will stumble at times, together we can do this. It truly does take a village.

Remember, no matter what any well-intentioned person tells you as to what to do with your baby's sleep . . . you have the final say! You are learning to be your baby's expert!

# Notes

1. "John Watson," Good Therapy, last modified July 13, 2015, https://www .goodtherapy.org/famous-psychologists/john-watson.html.

2. Margot Sunderland, *The Science of Parenting: How Today's Brain Research Can Help You Raise Happy, Emotionally Balanced Children* (New York: DK Publishing, 2006), 38.

3. Pamela S. Douglas and Peter S. Hill, "Behavioral Sleep Interventions in the First Six Months of Life Do Not Improve Outcomes for Mothers or Infants: A Systematic Review," *Journal of Developmental and Behavioral Pediatrics* 34, no. 7 (2013): 497–507.

4. "Erik Erikson," Good Therapy, last modified July 27, 2015, https://www .goodtherapy.org/famous-psychologists/erik-erikson.html.

5. Erin Olson, "Mirror Neurons and Mindful Parenting," *Flourish Consulting Milwaukee,* March 28, 2016, http://flourishcounselingmilwaukee.com /mirror-neurons-and-mindful-parenting/.

6. Oscar Serrallach, *The Postnatal Depletion Cure: A Complete Guide to Rebuilding Your Health and Reclaiming Your Energy for Mothers of Newborns, Toddlers, and Young Children* (Australia: Hachette, 2018), 32.

7. K. J. Saudino, "Behavioral Genetics and Child Temperament," *Journal of Developmental and Behavioral Pediatrics* 26, no. 3 (2005), 214–23. https://doi .org/10.1097/00004703-200506000-00010

8. A. Thomas and S. Chess, "The New York Longitudinal Study: From Infancy to Early Adult Life," in *The Study of Temperament: Changes, Continuities,*

*and Challenges,* ed. R. Plomin and J. Dunn (Mahwah, NJ: Erlbaum, 1986), 39–52.

9. Diana Divecha, "How Cosleeping Can Help You and Your Baby," *Greater Good Magazine,* February 7, 2020, https://greatergood.berkeley.edu/article /item/how_cosleeping_can_help_you_and_your_baby.

10. James J. McKenna, *Safe Infant Sleep: Experts Answer Your Cosleeping Questions* (Washington, DC: Platypus Media, 2020), 163.

11. Jodi Mindell, *Sleep Deprived No More: From Pregnancy to Early Motherhood— Helping You and Your Baby Sleep Through the Night* (New York: Marlow, 2007), 23.

12. Sunderland, *The Science of Parenting,* 48.

13. Sunderland, *The Science of Parenting,* 48.

14. Carmen W. H. Chan, Bernard M. H. Law, Yun-Hong Liu, et al., "The Association between Maternal Stress and Childhood Eczema: A Systematic Review," *International Journal of Environmental Research and Public Health* 15, no. 3 (2018): 395. https://doi.org/10.3390/ijerph15030395

15. Serrallach, *The Postnatal Depletion Cure,* 5.

16. Charles H. Zeanah, Jr., ed., *Handbook of Infant Mental Health,* 4th ed. (New York: Guildford Press, 2019), 26–27.

17. Zeanah, *Handbook of Infant Mental Health,* 26–27.

18. Sunderland, *The Science of Parenting,* 21.

19. Sunderland, *The Science of Parenting,* 18–19.

20. Sunderland, *The Science of Parenting,* 22.

21. Sunderland, *The Science of Parenting,* 21.

22. "First Month: Physical Appearance and Growth," *Healthy Children,* August 1, 2009, https://www.healthychildren.org/English/ages-stages/baby/Pages /First-Month-Physical-Appearance-and-Growth.aspx.

23. American Academy of Pediatrics, *Caring for Your Baby and Young Child: Birth to Age 5,* 7th ed. (New York: Bantam Books, 2019), 161.

24. American Academy of Pediatrics, *Caring for Your Baby and Young Child,* 161.

25. American Academy of Pediatrics, *Caring for Your Baby and Young Child,* 161.

26. T. Berry Brazelton, *Touchpoints: Birth to Three: Your Child's Emotional and Behavioral Development* (Cambridge: De Capo Press, 2006), 27.

27. American Academy of Pediatrics, *Caring for Your Baby and Young Child,* 161.

28. Brazelton, *Touchpoints,* 62.

29. William A. H. Sammons, *The Self-Calmed Baby: A Revolutionary New Approach to Parenting Your Infant* (Canada: Little Brown, 1989).

30. World Health Organization, *Infant and Young Child Feeding Handout* (2009).

31. Sanjeev Jain, "How Much and How Often Should Your Baby Eat?," *Healthy Children*, May 12, 2022, https://www.healthychildren.org/English/ages -stages/baby/feeding-nutrition/Pages/How-Often-and-How-Much-Should -Your-Baby-Eat.aspx.

32. World Health Organization, *Infant and Young Child Feeding Handout*.

33. World Health Organization, *Infant and Young Child Feeding Handout*.

34. Priscilla Dunstan, *Calm the Crying Using the Dunstan Baby Language: The Secret Baby Language That Reveals the Hidden Meaning behind an Infant's Cry* (New York: Avery, 2012), 40.

35. Dunstan, *Calm the Crying*, 40.

36. Jenifer R. Lightdale, David A. Gremse, Leo A. Heitlinger, et al., "Gastro-esophageal Reflux: Management Guidance for the Pediatrician," *Pediatrics* 131, no. 5 (2013): e1684–e1695. https://doi.org/10.1542/peds.2013-0421

37. Laura E. Berk, *Child Development,* 7th ed. (Boston: Allyn & Bacon, 2015).

38. S. Myruski, O. Gulyayeva, S. Birk, et al., "Digital Disruption? Maternal Mobile Device Use Is Related to Infant Social-Emotional Functioning," *Developmental Science* 21, no. 4 (2018): e12610. https://doi.org/10.1111/desc .12610

39. D. M. Teti, B. R. Kim, G. Mayer, et al., "Maternal Emotional Availability at Bedtime Predicts Infant Sleep Quality," *Journal of Family Psychology* 24, no. 3 (2010): 307–15.

40. Sunderland, *The Science of Parenting*, 46.

41. World Health Organization, *Infant and Young Child Feeding Handout*.

42. Sunderland, *The Science of Parenting*, 24.

43. Sunderland, *The Science of Parenting*, 36–37.

44. Sunderland, *The Science of Parenting*, 38.

45. Douglas Davies, *Child Development: A Practitioner's Guide* (Connecticut: Guilford, 1999). Allan N. Schore, *Affect dysregulation and disorders of the self* (New York: W.W. Norton & Company, 2003). E. Z. Tronick, "Emotions and Emotional Communication in Infants," *American Psychologist* 44 (1989): 112–119.

46. Sharla Kostelyk, "Calming Your Child's Fight, Flight or Freeze Response," *The Chaos and the Clutter,* https://www.thechaosandtheclutter.com/archives/helping-child-fight-flight-freeze-mode.

47. Harvey Karp, *The Happiest Baby Guide to Great Sleep: Simple Solutions for Kids from Birth to 5 Years* (New York: William Morrow, 2012), 180.

48. Patti Ideran and Mark Fishbein, *The CALM Baby Method: Solutions for Fussy Days and Sleepless Nights* (Itasca, IL: American Academy of Pediatrics, 2020), 152.

49. U.S. Department of Agriculture Food and Nutrition Service, "Getting to Know Your 2–8-Week-Old," *Baby Behavior* (2015).

50. Ideran and Fishbein, *The CALM Baby Method,* 39.

51. Dunstan, *Calm the Crying Using the Dunstan Baby Language,* 36.

52. Mayo Clinic, "Colic," https://www.mayoclinic.org/diseases-conditions/colic/symptoms-causes/syc-20371074.

53. Brazelton, *Touchpoints,* 63.

54. Brazelton, *Touchpoints,* 63.

55. Brazelton, *Touchpoints,* 63.

56. N. Razaz, W. T. Boyce, M. Brownell, et al., "Five-Minute Apgar Score as a Marker for Developmental Vulnerability at 5 Years of Age," *Archives of Disease in Childhood. Fetal and Neonatal Edition* 101, no. 2 (2016): F114–20.

57. Brazelton, *Touchpoints,* 59.

58. U.S. Department of Agriculture Food and Nutrition Service, "Getting to Know Your 2–8-Week-Old."

59. B. C. Galland, R. M. Sayers, S. L. Cameron, et al., "Anticipatory Guidance to Prevent Infant Sleep Problems within a Randomized Controlled Trial: Infant, Maternal, and Partner Outcomes at 6 Months of Age," *BMJ Open* 7, no. 5 (2017): e014908.

60. O. G. Jenni and M. A. Carskadon, "Normal Human Sleep at Different Ages: Infants to Adolescents," *Basics of Sleep Guide,* Sleep Research Society, (2005): 11–19.

61. Dunstan, *Calm the Crying Using the Dunstan Baby Language,* 34.

62. B. Caravale, S. Sette, E. Cannoni, et al., "Sleep Characteristics and Temperament in Preterm Children at Two Years of Age," *Journal of Clinical Sleep Medicine* 13, no. 9 (2017): 1081–88.

63. Serrallach, *The Postnatal Depletion Cure*, 32.

64. Tiffany Phu, Andrew Erhart, Pilyoung Kim, et al., "Two Open Windows, Part II: New Research on Infant and Caregiver Neurobiologic Change," (Aspen Institute, 2021). https://ascend-resources.aspeninstitute .org/resources/two-open-windows-ii-new-research-on-infant-and-caregiver -neurobiologic-change/.

65. Phu et al., "Two Open Windows."

66. Meredith Wadman, "Pregnancy Resculpts Women's Brains for at Least 2 Years," *Science*, December 16, 2016, https://www.science.org/content/article /pregnancy-resculpts-women-s-brains-least-2-years.

67. Serrallach, *The Postnatal Depletion Cure*, 4.

68. Serrallach, *The Postnatal Depletion Cure*, 5.

69. Serrallach, *The Postnatal Depletion Cure*, 32.

70. Serrallach, *The Postnatal Depletion Cure*, 97.

71. E. Abraham, T. Hendler, I. Shapira-Lichter, et al., "Father's Brain Is Sensitive to Childcare Experiences," *Proceedings of the National Academy of Sciences*, 111, no. 27 (2014): 9,792–97. https://doi.org/10.1073/pnas.1402569111

72. S. L. Mott, C. E. Schiller, J. G. Richards, et al., "Depression and Anxiety among Postpartum and Adoptive Mothers," *Archives of Women and Mental Health* 14, no. 4 (2011): 335–43.

73. Derek O'Neill and Jennifer Waldburger, *Calm Mama, Happy Baby: The Simple, Intuitive Way to Tame Tears, Improve Sleep, and Help Your Family Thrive* (Deerfield Beach: Health Communications, 2013), 29.

74. O'Neill and Waldburger, *Calm Mama Happy Baby*, 29.

75. Serrallach, *The Postnatal Depletion Cure*, 118.

76. Serrallach, *The Postnatal Depletion Cure*, 110.

77. Brazelton, *Touchpoints*.

78. Hetty van de Rijt and Frans Plooij, *The Wonder Weeks* (Netherlands: Kitty World Publishing, 2013), 47.

79. van de Rijt and Plooij, *The Wonder Weeks*, 47.

80. Ideran and Fishbein, *The CALM Baby Method*, 64.

81. Ideran and Fishbein, *The CALM Baby Method*, 64.

82. Brazelton, *Touchpoints*, 66.

83. Sunderland, *The Science of Parenting*, 46.

84. Warwick, "Research Says Massage May Help Infants Sleep More, Cry Less and Be Less Stressed," (2006).

85. Sammons, *The Self-Calmed Baby*, 81.

86. Mary Sheedy Kurcinka, *Raising Your Spirited Baby: A Breakthrough Guide to Thriving When Your Baby is More . . . Alert and Intense and Struggles to Sleep* (New York: William Morrow, 2010), 3.

87. Kurcinka, *Raising Your Spirited Baby*, 39–42.

88. Kurcinka, *Raising Your Spirited Baby*, 3.

89. Kurcinka, *Raising Your Spirited Baby*, 4.

90. Kurcinka, *Raising Your Spirited Baby*, 36–38.

91. S. J. Webb, C. S. Monk, and C. A. Nelson, "Mechanisms of Postnatal Neurobiological Development: Implications for Human Development," *Developmental Neuropsychology* 19 (2) (2001): 147–171. https://doi.org/10.1207/S15326942DN1902_2

92. M. Heimann, "Regression Periods in Human Infancy: An Introduction," in M. Heimann (ed.), *Regression Periods in Human Infancy* (2003), 1–6. A. Schore, "The Experience-Dependent Maturation of a Regulatory System in the Orbital Prefrontal Cortex and the Origin of Developmental Psychopathology," *Development and Psychopathology* 8 (1996): 59–87.

93. Jodi A. Mindell and Judith A. Owens, *A Clinical Guide to Pediatric Sleep: Diagnosis and Management of Sleep Problems*, 3rd ed. (Philadelphia: Wolters Kluwer, 2015), 22.

94. Mindell and Owens, *A Clinical Guide to Pediatric Sleep*, 22.

95. Serrallach, *The Postnatal Depletion Cure*, 110.

96. O'Neill and Waldburger, *Calm Mama, Happy Baby*, 38–39.

97. Anna Davies, "Are You Guilty of Maternal Gatekeeping?" *The Bump*, December 17, 2017, https://www.thebump.com/a/maternal-gatekeeping.

98. Brazelton, *Touchpoints*, 62.

99. van de Rijt and Plooij, *The Wonder Weeks*, 83.

100. Brazelton, *Touchpoints*, 75.

101. Ideran and Fishbein, *The CALM Baby Method*, 29–30.

102. Colleen de Bellefonds, "Thumb-Sucking Baby: Is It Okay for Newborns to Suck Their Thumbs?" *What to Expect*, September 1, 2022, https://www.whattoexpect.com/first-year/ask-heidi/thumb-sucking-baby.aspx.

103. W. Thomas Boyce, *The Orchid and the Dandelion: Why Sensitive Children Face Challenges and How All Can Thrive* (New York, Knopf: 2019).

104. Serrallach, *The Postnatal Depletion Cure*, 241.

105. "Vitamin D Benefits," *Healthline,* https://www.healthline.com/health/food -nutrition/benefits-vitamin-d.

106. van de Rijt and Plooij, *The Wonder Weeks*, 120.

107. van de Rijt and Plooij, *The Wonder Weeks*, 110.

108. van de Rijt and Plooij, *The Wonder Weeks*, 129.

109. van de Rijt and Plooij, *The Wonder Weeks*, 120.

110. Danielle Pacheco, "How Your Baby's Sleep Cycle Differs from Your Own," *Sleep Foundation,* updated March 11, 2022, https://www.sleepfoundation .org/baby-sleep/baby-sleep-cycle.

111. Brazelton, *Touchpoints*, 94.

112. Brazelton, *Touchpoints,* 95.

113. A. Thomas and S. Chess, "The New York Longitudinal Study: From Infancy to Early Adult Life," in *The Study of Temperament: Changes, Continuities, and Challenges,* ed. R. Plomin and J. Dunn (Mahwah, NJ: Erlbaum, 1986), 39–52.

114. van de Rijt and Plooij, *The Wonder Weeks,* 464.

115. SpoonfulONE, "How it Works," SpoonfulONE.com.

116. Marc Weissbluth, *Healthy Sleep Habits, Happy Child,* (New York: Ballantine, 1987), 53.

117. Erin Olson, "Mirror Neurons and Mindful Parenting," *Flourish Counseling Milwaukee,* March 28, 2016, http://flourishcounselingmilwaukee.com /mirror-neurons-and-mindful-parenting/.

# Index

**A**

AAP. *see* American Academy of
    Pediatrics
accidental co-sleepers, 40
active/fussy babies
    about, 212
    sleep strategies for, 212–213
active sleep, 97–98. *see also* REM sleep
activity level, 33
acupressure, 88
acupuncture, 87, 114, 190
adaptability, 33
adjusted age, 107
adoption, 42
adrenaline, 53
age, adjusted, 107
Agrawal, Radha, 14, 47–48, 110
alert babies. *see also* active/fussy babies
    about, 32, 92–93
    "cry it out" method with, 213
    in second month, 138–140
    sleep coaching, 214, 247–248
    sleep shaping with, 172–174
    supporting, 94, 139–140, 174–175
    Switcheroo technique with, 184
allergies, 19, 69, 86, 241

American Academy of Pediatrics (AAP),
    36, 37, 56, 62, 83, 206, 240
"and," as term, 232
Ann (parent), 9, 193–194
anxiety
    and PMADs, 112
    during sleep coaching, 259
    stranger, 196, 237, 238–239,
        245–246
    stranger vs. separation, 239
appetite, 201
approach/withdrawal, 33
arousal, 92, 139
*A soñar,* 13
assess (SOAR), 21
attachment
    about, 6, 28–30
    bonding with baby, 29–30
    fifth month, 243
    first month, 71–77
    fourth month, 204
    pre-birth, 28–30
    second month, 128–129
    and temperament, 247
    third month, 167–168
attachment parenting, 71

**B**
baby blues, 111–112
"baby brain," 108–109
baby bundle, 84
baby holds, 84
Baby-Led Sleep Coaching
    at bedtime only (phase 1), 259–263
    and communication between
        parents, 231–232
    at five months, 252–273
    Modified Shuffle (*see* Modified
        Shuffle)
    phases of, 258
    readiness checklist, 222–223
    transitioning to, 222–223
    trust during, 243
Baby-Led Sleep Shaping
    about, 7
    first month, 104–106
    in first month, 104
    in second month, 145
    in third month and beyond, 178
    transitioning from, 224–230
Baby-Led Sleep Shaping and
    Coaching™, 182–183, 226–227,
    256–257
    about, 21–24
    at 4 months, 218
    modifying, 186
    soothing in, 30
bad habits
    creating, 96, 216
    during 4-month sleep regression,
        217
Ball, Helen, 39
Barr, Ronald, 122–123
bedsharing. *see* co-sleeping
bedtime
    during Baby-Led Sleep Coaching
        (phase 1), 260
    beginning a, 186

earlier, 179–180
emotional availability at, 74
at 4 months, 217
regulating, 218
routines for, 76, 101–102, 159
bedtime only coaching (phase 1 of
    Baby-Led Sleep Coaching),
    259–263
behaviorism, 3–4
Bennett, Shoshana, 15, 28–29
    on bonding, 72–73
    on expectations, 95
    on myths of parenthood, 153
    on parental sleep, 149
    on PMADs, 43, 45, 112
    on trauma, 31
*Beyond the Blues* (Bennett), 15
Biel, Lindsey, 13, 107
bipolar disorder, 111
bird feeders, 51
birth mothers, maternal-fetal
    attachment with, 29
birth plan, 44–45
birth to 4 months. *see* first month
birth weight, 55
"blackout sleep," 47
body contact. *see* touch
body feeling technique, 152
bonding
    in first month, 72–73
    and skin-to-skin contact, 77
    strategies for, 74–75
bottle feeding, 65–66
bottle refusal, 166
Boyce, W. Thomas, 171
brain
    changes in parental, 8, 109
    development of, 53–55
        second, 121
    emotional, 53–54
    during meditation, 47

Brazelton, T. Berry, 90, 91
breastfeeding
    and cluster feeding, 128
    and colic, 87
    and eczema, 90
    issues with, 68–69
    planning your nights for, 42
    and return to work, 293
breastmilk, 61, 124
breathing, 133, 152
The Bump website, 154
burnout, 232
"but," replacing, 232

**C**

The CALM Baby Method, 169
*The Calm Baby Method* (Ideran and
    Fishbein), 129
"calm but awake"
    defined, 253
    with rocked/held/walked to sleep
        babies, 261
Calming Breath (exercise), 152
*Calm Mama, Happy Baby* (O'Neill and
    Waldburger), 113, 152
"can't," 233
caregivers, 295
*Caring for Your Baby* (AAP), 56
catnaps, 176
cause and effect, 196, 238
cell phone use, 72–73
cereal, 202
childcare workers, 109
circadian rhythms
    in Baby-Led Sleep Coaching (phase
        1), 261
    in first month, 100
    schedules to support, 159
    in second month, 143
    supporting, 218
    in third month, 175–176

cluster feeding, 127–128
cognitive awareness, 195
colic, 207
    case example of, 88–89
    causes of, 86–87
    soothing, 86, 170
    soothing during, 210
    treating, 87–88
committed co-sleepers, 40
communication, between parents,
    231–232
conflict provoking words, 232
confusion, day-night, 100
cortisol, 53, 133, 141, 179
co-sleeping, 38–41
    about, 38–39
    accidental, 40
    with alert babies, 95
    committed, 40
    in first month, 104–105
    at 4 months, 230
    reactive, 41
    in second month, 148
    short-term, 40
    in third month, 187
    transitioning from, 148–149
    types of, 39–40
cow's milk, 86
CPSC (U.S. Consumer Product Safety
    Commission), 38
Cradle Company, 12
crying
    common causes of, 130–131
    early infant, 122
    first month, 57
    in first month, 57
    prolonged, 78, 259
    during sensations leap, 121
    during sleep coaching, 258–259
"cry it out" method, 4, 141, 213, 222
C-sections, 36

cuddling, 74, 76–77
cues
    hunger, 66–68
    learning, 20
    reading temperament, 93
    sleep, 94, 103–104, 205
    social, 245

**D**
dairy, 70
dandelions. *see* non-alert babies
Daybreaker, 14, 47–48
daycare, 164, 295–296
day-night confusion, 100
deep breathing, 152
deep sleep, 98–99
delivery wish list, 44–45
depletion, postnatal, 189
depression, 111
depth perception, 195
development
    and bonding, 29–30
    brain, 53–55
    crying, 57
    fifth month, 237–240
    first month, 53–60
    fourth month, 195–201
    fourth trimester, 58
    habituation, 57–58
    newborn reflexes, 56–57
    psychological, 6
    second month, 120–123
    and sleep regression, 197
    supporting, for better sleep, 58–59
    third month, 160–162
    variability in, 17–18
dexterity, 238
Diaz, Natalie, 18
difficult babies. *see* active/fussy babies
distracted feeding, 165–166
distractibility, 33

distractions, for soothing, 134
DOSE, 48
Douglas, Pamela, 5
downstairs brain, 53–54
dream feed, 143–144, 163–164, 203
drool, 210
Dunstan, Priscilla, 68
Dunstan Baby Language, 68, 85, 104
dysregulation, 55–56, 292

**E**
easy and flexible babies, 211, 212
eczema
    case example of, 235–236
    and prolonged maternal stress, 43
    soothing, 90, 170
EFT, 48
8 to 12 weeks. *see* third month
Emily (parent), 9, 117–119
emotional availability, 73–74
Emotional Availability Scales, 73–74
emotional brain, 53–54
engagement, with alert babies, 173
Erikson, Erik, 6
Escalante, Alison, 15, 45
expectations, 95, 140–141
extinction method, 3–4
eye contact, 72–73

**F**
facial expressions, 85, 204
fantasy temperament, 33
FAST (feeding, attachment, soothing, temperament), 6–7, 18–20
Federal Patient Protection and Affordable Care Act (2010), 294–295
feeding
    about, 6
    additional, during 4-month sleep regression, 216

bottle, 65–66
challenges to (*see* feeding challenges)
cluster, 127–128
distracted, 165–166
dream, 143–144, 163–164, 203
fifth month, 240–243
first month, 60–71
fourth month, 201–204
mother's, 27–28
mother's pre-birth, 27–28
on-demand, 62, 63
on-demand vs. scheduled, 63–65
routines for, 75
second month, 123–128
to sleep, 260
supporting sleep through, 62–63
third month, 162–167
feeding, attachment, soothing,
    temperament (FAST), 6–7, 18–20
feeding challenges
  in first month, 68–69
  at five months, 242
  at 4 months, 204
  in second month, 125–128
  in third month, 165–167
feeding logs, 64, 242
feeding strikes, 242
feelings, handling, 46–48
fifth month, 235–289
  attachment, 243
  development, 237–240
  feeding, 240–243
  parental self-care, 287–288
  sleep, 249–286
  soothing, 243–246
  temperament, 246–248
First Candle, 37
first month, 51–116
  attachment, 71–77
  baby-led sleep shaping, 104–106
  brain development, 53–55

crying, 57
development, 53–60
feeding, 60–71
fourth trimester, 58
habituation, 57–58
newborn reflexes, 56–57
parental self-care, 108–115
premature birth, 106–108
returning home during, 52–53
sleep, 96–104
soothing, 77–91
temperament, 91–95
tummy time, 59–60
Fishbein, Mark, 129
Fletcher, Emily, 15, 46–47, 151, 189
flexibility, 45–46, 120
food
  sensitivities to, 87
foods
  intolerances to, 86
  solid, 202, 241
"football" hold, 84
formula
  and colic, 87
  in first month, 70–71
  first month average intake, 61
  second month average intake, 124
"four in/seven out" breathing
    technique, 114
4-month sleep regression
  about, 195–199
  case example of, 235–236
  getting through, 216
fourth month, 193–234
  attachment, 204
  development, 195–201
  feeding, 201–204
  parental self-care, 231–233
  sleep, 215–230
  soothing, 204–210
  temperament, 211–215

fourth trimester, 58
4 to 8 weeks. *see* second month
frustration, 292
fussiness
    and hunger cues, 67
    soothing during, 205
    during tummy time, 200

**G**
gassy babies, 83
genetics, 33
Gentle Sleep Coaches, 9, 11–16
GERD (gastroesophageal reflux
    disease)
    in second month, 126
    signs of, 69
    soothing during, 170, 210
    tactics to use during, 70
goodbye routines, 246
goodness of fit, 34
Gordon, Macall
    about, 12
    on alert babies, 94, 171–173, 214
    on attachment, 128, 167
    on "cry it out" method, 222
    on readiness for sleep coaching, 221
Gorman, Amanda, 44
graduated extinction method, 3
Grandin, Temple, 13
grasp, pincer, 238
Green, Robin Ray, 87, 114
green zone, 139
Guarneri, Mimi, 114

**H**
habituation
    in first month, 57–58, 105–106
    in second month, 136–137
*Handbook of Infant Mental Health,* 48
*The Happiest Baby on the Block* (Karp),
    79

Healthy Child Concierge, 14
Healthy Kids Happy Kids, 13–14
hemorrhages, 31
holds, baby, 84
holistic therapies, 88
home, returning, 52–53
hormones, 186
    and circadian rhythms, 100
    and parental self-care, 8, 24
    and PMADs, 111
Horn, Sam, 16, 232
hunger cues, 66–68
hyperpresence, 190

**I**
Ideran, Patti, 129
intensity, of alert babies, 33, 172–173
interactions, for bonding, 72–73
interactive repairs, 167
Intrigue Agency, 16
irregularity, in alert babies, 173–174
Irvine, Heather
    about, 11–12
    on dream feed, 163–164, 220
    on 4-month regression, 242
    on latch challenges, 126
    on pacifiers, 206
    on return to work, 293

**J**
jaundice, 51
Jiggle and Soothe, 184–185
Jiggle and Soothe 2.0, 224, 229–230
Joanne (parent), 235–236
Jordan, Brandi, 12, 162, 166, 293
Joy Practice, 47–48, 110, 151

**K**
kangaroo care, 77
Karp, Harvey, 79, 82
Kurcinka, Mary Sheedy, 138–139

**L**
latch challenges, 125–126
light, natural, 219
Loizides, Anthony, 127

**M**
Mad to Glad Blueprint, 16
manifesting, 46
marathon feed. *see* cluster feeding
massages, 94, 120, 133
maternal gatekeeping, 153–154
Maven Clinic, 12
Mayo Clinic, 86
McKenna, James J., 38–39
meditation, 46–47, 151
melatonin, 159, 186
meltdowns, 137–138
mesh teething bags, 210
milestones, 17–18
milk
    breastmilk, 61, 124
    cow's, 86
    production of, 63–64
    soy, 86
    supply of (*see* milk supply)
milk supply
    and cluster feeding, 128
    decrease in, 201
    in third month, 166
Mindell, Jodi, 41
mindfulness, 46, 151, 189–190
Modified Shuffle, 229
    about, 252–253
    case example of, 236
    and feeding to sleep, 260
    guidelines for, 255
    with rocked/held/walked to sleep
        babies, 261
    steps for, 253–254
Moe, Samantha, 16, 53
Montessori-style sleep, 35

mood, 33
Moon Breath (exercise), 152
moro, 57, 79–80
Mother-Baby Sleep Laboratory, 38
mother's feeding, 27–28
movement
    parental, 151
    for soothing, 134
multitasks, 8

**N**
nannies, 109, 295–296
naps
    during Baby-Led Sleep Coaching
        (phase 1), 262
    daytime, 101
    extension strategies for, 263
    at 4 months, 219
    limiting, 144
    plan for, in Baby-Led Sleep
        Coaching (phase 1), 261–262
    power, 148
    routines for, 76, 102
    in second month, 142–143, 146
    in third month, 176
    and wakeful windows, 215
National Association of Birth Workers
    of Color, 12
National Center on Shaken Baby
    Syndrome (NCSBS), 122–123
natural light, 219
needs, responding to, 76
negative sleep association, 99
neocortex, 54
Neville, Helen, 32
newborn reflexes, 56–57
Newborns & Beyond, 12
*New England Journal of Medicine,* 202
Nicole (parent), 82
night sleep consolidation, 142,
    175–176

nighttime feedings
    doctor and lactation advice for, 220
    reducing, 220
    and solid foods, 202–203
    in third month, 164
nighttime sleep, lengthening, 143
night wakings, during Baby-Led Sleep
        Coaching (phase 1), 260
non-alert babies, 171
non-REM sleep, 98–99, 197
nursing strikes, 166
nutrition, 27–28. *see also* feeding

**O**
obesity, 202
object permanence, 196, 237–238
observe (SOAR), 21
obsessive compulsive disorder, 111
"off-duty" hours, 189
on-demand feeding, 62, 63
O'Neill, Derek, 113–114, 152
*The Orchid and the Dandelion* (Boyce),
    171
orchids. *see* alert babies
overfeeding, 241
overstimulation, 90–91, 108
    cues for, 137
    preventing, 145, 218
    in second month, 135–136
overtiredness, 146–147, 179–180
oxytocin, 77

**P**
pacifiers
    in first month, 83–84
    at 4 months, 205–207
    "pacifier-holding" products, 206
    in second month, 131–132
    and stranger anxiety, 245
    during teething, 210
    weaning from, 207

panic disorder, 111
parental self-care
    and brain development, 108–109
    and delivery wish list, 44
    fifth month, 287–288
    first month, 108–115
    fourth month, 231–233
    handling "big feelings," 46
    importance of, 7–8, 24–25, 43
    joy practice, 47–48
    meditation, 46–47
    and myths about parenthood,
        45–46, 153–155
    pre-birth, 43–48
    prioritizing, 44
    second month, 150–155
    sleep for, 41–42
    third month, 189–191
parental sleep, 41–42
parent-child bond. *see* attachment
patience, 230
Paynel, Jeanne-Marie, 35
pediatric acupuncture, 87
pelvic floor exercises, 190
Pennsylvania State University, 73
perceptiveness, 173
"the Period of PURPLE Crying,"
        122–123, 130
persistence, 33, 173
pincer grasp, 238
pituitary gland, 77
playtime, routines for, 75
"please," 233
Plooij, Frans, 121
PMADs. *see* postpartum mood and
        anxiety disorders
poop, 62
postnatal depletion, 189
*The Postnatal Depletion Cure*
        (Serrallach), 8, 44, 109, 151
postpartum bipolar disorder, 111

postpartum depletion, 109–110

postpartum depression, 111

*Postpartum Depression for Dummies*
(Bennett), 15

postpartum mood and anxiety
disorders (PMADs)

baby blues vs., 111–112

at 4 months, 230

planning for, 43

in third month, 189

postpartum obsessive compulsive
disorder, 111

postpartum panic disorder, 111

postpartum post-traumatic stress
disorder, 111

postpartum psychosis, 111

post-traumatic stress disorder (PTSD),
31, 111

power naps, 148

"practice week," 294

pre-bed routines, 205

pre-birth, 27–49

attachment, 28–30

mother's feeding, 27–28

mother's sleep, 34–43

parental self-care, 43–48

soothing, 30–32

temperament, 32–34

predictability, 74–75, 159

*Pregnant on Prozac and Children of the
Depressed* (Bennett), 15

premature babies

about, 18, 106–107

adjusted age in, 107

in first month, 106–108

sensory processing in, 107

sleep coaching readiness in, 249

tip for helping, 108

pre-sleep coaching techniques, 181–185

prolactin, 77

prolonged crying, 78, 259

prolonged maternal stress, 43

psychological development, 6

psychosis, 111

pumping, 294–295

PURPLE crying, 122–123

**R**

*Raising a Sensory Smart Child* (Biel),
13, 107

*Raising your Spirited Baby* (Kurcinka),
138

rapid eye movement (REM), 98

reactive co-sleeping, 41

reassurance, verbal, 255

red zone, 139

reflex(es)

newborn, 56–57

tongue-thrust, 241

reflux

case example of, 235–236

and colic, 86

in first month, 69–70

and pacifiers, 207

in second month, 126

regurgitation. *see* reflux

relaxing visualizations, 151–152

REM (rapid eye movement), 98

REM sleep, 97–98, 197

respond (SOAR), 21

responding to needs, 76

returning home, 52–53

return to work, 164, 293–295

reunion routines, 246

reverse cycling, 166–167, 204, 242

rhythmicity, 33

rice cereal, 202

rocked to sleep, 261

rolling

attempts to, 196

back to front, 240

front to back, 240

rolling (*continued*)
  as self-soothing, 208, 239
  teaching your baby to, 201
  during tummy time, 200, 239–240
rollover feeding. *see* dream feed
room-darkening shades, 205
room sharing, 36–38
rooting about, 56
routines
  for attachment, 204
  benefits of, for whole family, 120
  for bonding, 74–76
  building trust through, 168
  goodbye, 246
  month 3 and beyond, 218
  pre-bed, 205
  reunion, 246
  in second month, 119–120, 145
  in third month and beyond, 178

**S**
*Safe Infant Sleep* (McKenna), 38
safety
  and co-sleeping, 40
  in fourth month, 195
  during kangaroo care, 77
  while swaddling, 80
scheduled feeding
  in first month, 62–64
  introducing, 162–163
  in second month, 124–125
schedules. *see also* routines
  introducing, 158–159
  for parental self-care, 190–191
  third month, 158–159
second month, 117–156
  attachment, 128–129
  development, 120–123
  feeding, 123–128
  parental self-care, 150–155
  routines during, 119–120

  sleep, 140–150
  soothing, 129–138
  temperament, 138–140
self-care, parental. *see* parental self-care
self-regulation, 2, 55
self-soothing
  development of, 7, 208–209
  and extinction method, 4
  in month five, 244
  in third month, 160–161
senses, soothing through, 132
sensory processing
  in premature babies, 107
  in second month, 121
*Sensory Processing Challenges* (Biel), 13
sensory threshold, 33
separation anxiety, 239
Serrallach, Oscar
  on baby brain, 109
  on parental movement, 151
  on parental self-care, 44, 47–48
  on postnatal brain development, 8
  on postnatal depletion, 189
  on postpartum depletion, 110
  on stress management, 114
shades, room-darkening, 205
short-term co-sleepers, 40
"shoulds," 232
"ShouldStorm," 45
"The Should Storm" (Escalante), 15
shushing, 82
shy/cautious babies. *see* slow-to-warm
  babies
side car, 38
side holding, 81–82
SIDS. *see* Sudden Infant Death
  Syndrome
Siegel, Daniel, 29, 53
SIESTA (Study of Infants' Emergent
  Sleep Trajectories), 73–74
*Sigh, See, Start* (Escalante), 45

silicone toothbrushes, 210
16 to 20 weeks. *see* fifth month
sixth month, 292
skin-to-skin contact, 77
sleep
  challenges with (*see* sleep challenges)
  fifth month, 249–286
  first month, 96–104
  fourth month, 215–230
  Montessori-style, 35
  mother's pre-birth, 34–43
  parental, 41–42, 149–150
  room sharing, 36–38
  second month, 140–150
  states of, 97–99
  Sudden Infant Death Syndrome
    (SIDS), 36–37
  third month, 175–189
sleep challenges
  in first month, 105
  in third month, 187–189
sleep coaching
  defined, 3
  early, 221
  feeding during, 240
  methods for, 224
  and parental self-care, 231
  readiness for, 220–223, 249–252
  sleep shaping vs., 224
  waiting for, 177
sleep crutches, 99, 181
sleep cues, 94, 103–104, 205
sleep cycles, changes in, 197
*Sleep Deprived No More* (Mindell), 41
sleep-friendly environments, 34–35,
    102–103, 218
*The Sleep Lady's Good Night Sleep Tight*
    (Sleep Lady), 2, 252
Sleep Lady Shuffle, 252
sleep logs, 64
sleep regression

case example, 197–199
  at 4 months (*see* 4-month sleep
    regression)
sleep shaping
  defined, 3
  in first month, 100
  sleep coaching vs., 224
sleep training
  defined, 3
  waiting for, 177
slow-to-warm babies
  about, 212
  sleep strategies for, 212
smell(s)
  development of, 160
  soothing, 134–135
smiles, 168
snacking, 243
SOAR (stop, observe, assess, and
    respond)
  about, 20–21, 30
  with alert babies, 140
  and on-demand feeding, 65
  for soothing, 209–210
social cues, 245
social media, 110
solid foods, 202, 241
*SOMEDAY is Not a Day in the Week*
    (Horn), 16
Song, Elisa, 13–14, 69, 87–88
soothing
  about, 6–7
  additional, during 4-month sleep
    regression, 216
  challenges to (*see* soothing
    challenges)
  cues for, 84–85
  experimenting with, 129
  fifth month, 243–246
  first month, 77–91
  fourth month, 204–210

soothing (*continued*)
    importance of, 96
    during Modified Shuffle, 255
    pre-birth, 30–32
    second month, 129–138
    third month, 168–170
    through senses, 132
    tips for, 79–84, 131, 169
soothing challenges
    in fifth month, 245–246
    in first month, 85–91
    in fourth month, 210–211
    in second month, 135–138
    in third month, 170
sounds, soothing, 134–135
soy milk, 86
spirited babies. *see* alert babies
spitting up. *see* reflux
startle, 57, 79–80
stop (SOAR), 20
stop, observe, assess, and respond
    (SOAR). *see* SOAR
stranger anxiety, 196, 237, 238–239,
    245–246
stress
    and massage, 133
    and meditation, 47
    effects of parental, 43
    parental, 113–114
    prolonged, 43
strikes
    feeding, 242
    nursing, 166
Study of Infants' Emergent Sleep
    Trajectories (SIESTA), 73–74
sucking, 56, 83
Sudden Infant Death Syndrome
    (SIDS)
    and pacifiers, 206
    and room sharing, 36–37

    and side holding, 82
    and tummy time, 59
Super Slow Shuffle, 224–229, 255, 261
swaddling
    about, 79–81
    alternatives to, 81
    benefits of, 81
    with premature babies, 108
    and rolling, 240
    weaning from, 188–189
swinging, 82–83, 134
Switcheroo technique, 181–184

**T**
taste, development of, 160
teething, 210
teething bags, mesh, 210
temperament
    about, 7
    and arousal, 92
    characteristics of, 33
    defined, 32
    early markers of, 91
    fantasy, 33
    fifth month, 246–248
    first month, 91–95
    fourth month, 211–215
    and goodness of fit, 34
    molding, 247
    pre-birth, 32–34
    second month, 138–140
    supporting your baby's, 93
    third month, 170–175
    types of, 211–215
*Temperament Tools* (Neville), 32
Temple, Ana-Maria, 14, 28, 44, 90,
    210
terminology, reducing conflict
    provoking, 232
Teti, Douglas, 73–74

therapies, holistic, 88
third month, 157–192
  attachment, 167–168
  development, 160–162
  feeding, 162–167
  parental self-care, 189–191
  schedules, 158–159
  sleep, 175–189
  soothing, 168–170
  temperament, 170–175
"three Cs," 121
3pm rule, 89
thumb sucking, 169, 244–245
tongue and lip tie, 86
Tongue-Fu!, 232
*Tongue Fu!* (Horn), 16
tongue-thrust reflex, 241
toothbrushes, silicone, 210
touch
  with alert babies, 140
  importance of, 76–77
  during Modified Shuffle, 255
  skin-to-skin contact, 77
  soothing with, 132–133
*Touchpoints* (Brazelton), 90
transition plans, for return to work, 294–295
Tranter, Maryanne, 14, 86, 123
trauma, 31
trust
  and attachment, 243
  building, 141
  soothing to build, 79
  through routines, 168
tummy time
  about, 59
  alternative positions for, 59–60
  and GERD, 70
  in month five, 239–240
  at 4 months, 200–201
  in second month, 123
  in third month, 161
12 to 16 weeks. *see* fourth month
twins, 18
Tyler, Anne, 1

**U**
underfeeding, 241
University of Warwick, 133
unpredictability, 173–174
unsupported crying, 259
upstairs brain, 53–54
U.S. Consumer Product Safety Commission (CPSC), 38

**V**
van de Rijt, Hetty, 121
verbal reassurance, 255
vision, development of, 160

**W**
wakeful windows
  about, 215
  during Baby-Led Sleep Coaching (phase 1), 262
  in second month, 142–143
  swaddling during, 81
wake time
  at 4 months, 217
  regulating, 218
wake-up, regulating, 102
Waldburger, Jennifer, 113–114, 152
walking mindfulness, 189–190
Watson, John, 3–4, 32
weaning
  from swaddling, 188–189
  when to start, 132
weight, birth, 55
*What's Holding You Back* (Horn), 16
white noise, 82

Willow (case example), 197–199
withdrawal, 78
*The Wonder Weeks* (van de Rijt and
      Plooij), 121, 161, 196
"Words to Lose," 232
"Words to Use," 232
work, return to, 164, 293–295
World Health Organization, 60

**Y**
yellow zone, 139
*The Yes Brain* (Siegel), 29

**Z**
Zeanah, Charles, 48
Zepeda, Gabriela, 84
      about, 13
      on bottle feeding, 66
      on teething, 210
      on tummy time, 161
Ziva Meditation, 15, 46
Ziva Technique, 15

# About the Author

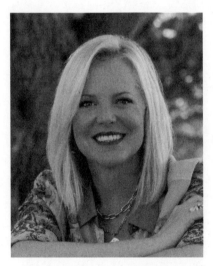

**Kim West, MSW**, is a mother of two daughters and a clinical social worker (a child and family therapist) for over 25 years. Known as The Sleep Lady® by her clients, she has personally helped over 20,000 tired parents all over the world get a good night's sleep without letting their children cry it out alone.

Kim has appeared on *Dr. Phil*, the *Today* show, *NBC Nightly News*, *Good Morning America*, TLC's *Bringing Home Baby*, and CNN, and has been written about in a number of publications including the *Wall Street Journal*, Associated Press, *Baby Talk*, *Parenting*, the *Baltimore Sun*, *USA Today*, the *Telegraph*, *The Irish Independent*, and the *Washington Post*.

Kim is the author of three books: *The Sleep Lady's Good Night, Sleep Tight: Gentle Proven Solutions to Help Your Child Sleep Well and Wake Up Happy*; *The Good Night, Sleep Tight Workbook*; and *The Good Night, Sleep Tight Workbook for Children with Special Needs*. Her first book, *The Sleep Lady's Good Night, Sleep Tight*, is in its third edition and has sold over 140,000 paperback copies.

Dedicated to providing tired parents with excellent sleep advice and coaching, she started the Gentle Sleep Coach® Training and Certification program in

2010—the first and most comprehensive pediatric sleep consultant training program in the world. This program was the start to what is now a global industry: baby and child sleep consultants. To date, the Gentle Sleep Coach Training and Certification program is available in two languages.

Her websites:

SleepLady.com
GentleSleepCoach.com

Follow her on:

Facebook: TheSleepLady
Pinterest: thesleeplady
Instagram: @thesleeplady

## WE WANT TO HEAR YOUR SUCCESS STORIES!

SleepLady.com/Testimonials

## INTERVIEW THE SLEEP LADY® FOR YOUR TV SHOW, PUBLICATION, OR PODCAST

SleepLady.com/Podcast

## LEARN ABOUT OUR ONLINE SLEEP COURSE FOR PARENTS AND CAREGIVERS OF 0–5-MONTH-OLDS

GentleNewbornSleep.com

## WORK WITH ONE OF OUR CERTIFIED GENTLE SLEEP COACHES OR BECOME ONE YOURSELF

To set up a consult with a Gentle Sleep Coach: FindaSleepCoach.com

To become a certified Gentle Sleep Coach: GentleSleepCoach.com